Internet of Medical Things

Internet of Medical Things

Paradigm of Wearable Devices

Edited by

*Manuel Cardona, Vijender Kumar Solanki,
and Cecilia E. García Cena*

CRC Press
Taylor & Francis Group
Boca Raton London New York

CRC Press is an imprint of the
Taylor & Francis Group, an **informa** business

First edition published 2021
by CRC Press
6000 Broken Sound Parkway NW, Suite 300, Boca Raton, FL 33487-2742
and by CRC Press
2 Park Square, Milton Park, Abingdon, Oxon, OX14 4RN

Library of Congress Cataloging-in-Publication Data

Names: Cardona, Manuel, 1934- editor. | Solanki, Vijender Kumar 1980- editor. | Cena, Cecilia E. García, editor.
Title: Internet of medical things : paradigm of wearable devices / edited by Manuel Cardona, Vijender Kumar Solanki, and Cecilia E. García Cena.
Description: First edition. | Boca Raton, FL : CRC Press, 2021. | Series: Internet of everything (ioe): security and privacy paradigm | Includes bibliographical references and index.
Identifiers: LCCN 2020038485 (print) | LCCN 2020038486 (ebook) | ISBN 9780367272630 (hardback) | ISBN 9780429296864 (ebook)
Subjects: LCSH: Medical technology. | Medical care--Technological innovations. | Medical informatics. | Data mining.
Classification: LCC R855.3 .I576 2021 (print) | LCC R855.3 (ebook) | DDC 610.285--dc23
LC record available at https://lccn.loc.gov/2020038485
LC ebook record available at https://lccn.loc.gov/2020038486

ISBN: 978-0-367-27263-0 (hbk)
ISBN: 978-0-429-29686-4 (ebk)

Typeset in Times
by KnowledgeWorks Global Ltd.

Contents

Preface vii
Editors xi
Contributors xiii

Chapter 1 Fundamentals and Paradigms in the Internet of Things 1
Claudia Lorena Garzón-Castro and Ramiro Velázquez

Chapter 2 Internet of Medical Things: Current and Future Trends 19
Lucia Alonso Virgos, Miguel A. Sanchez Vidales, Fernando López Hernández, and J. Javier Rainer Granados

Chapter 3 An Overview on Wearable Devices for Medical Applications 37
Meet Kumari and Meenu Gupta

Chapter 4 Blockchain-Based IoT for Personalized Pharmaceuticals 51
Rehab A. Rayan and Christos Tsagkaris

Chapter 5 Wearable/Implantable Devices for Monitoring Systems 63
Pawan Kumar and Shabana Urooj

Chapter 6 Wearable Sensors for Monitoring Exercise and Fatigue Estimation in Rehabilitation 83
Maria J. Pinto-Bernal, Andres Aguirre, Carlos A. Cifuentes, and Marcela Munera

Chapter 7 Conversational Agents for Healthcare Delivery: Potential Solutions to the Challenges of the Pandemic 111
Margarita Bautista, Carlos A. Cifuentes, and Marcela Munera

Chapter 8 Role of Big Data in e-Healthcare Application for Managing a Large Amount of Data 137
Meenu Gupta, Dr. Rachna Jain, Rachit Singhal, and Jaspreet Singh

Index 165

Preface

In Chapter 1, "Fundamentals and Paradigms in the Internet of Things," contributed by Claudia L. Garzón-Castro and Ramiro Velázquez, they discuss new technologies which have permeated all activities in daily life, leading to many objects being connected to and communicated through a network in one way or another. This connection of multiple components and devices through the Internet is known as the Internet of Things (IoT). The IoT helps to collect data from devices in real time, link devices with backend systems, ensure interoperability and build and operate diverse applications. Like most technological advancements, the aim of IoT is to offer the user comfort in various areas while being both time and cost effective. IoT has been used in several applications including, but not limited to, remote monitoring and telemetry for predictive maintenance. This diversity of applications has allowed the use of IoT in various fields of action such as: environmental and urban infrastructure control, mass production, health, transport systems, and the energy industry, among others. This chapter presents a holistic vision of the fundamentals of the IoT with the aim of providing a comprehensive overview to readers interested in the topic. The chapter addresses the most relevant concepts involved in the IoT such as architectures, sensors, actuators, storage, communication protocols, and user interfaces. Finally, some IoT-based development applications for healthcare were provided. In this sense, it can be concluded that IoT can be successfully used in services associated to patient monitoring, risky situations detection, and telemedicine, among other applications.

Chapter 2 is titled, "Internet of Medical Things: Current and Future Trends." The Internet of Medical Things (IoMT) establishes the necessary scenario for medical devices and applications to evolve through information technology. In this chapter, the authors, Lucia Alonso Virgos, Miguel A. Sanchez Vidales, Fernando López Hernández, and J. Javier Rainer Granados, analyze the most relevant current and future trends, referred to as IoMT. The objective of IoMT is to offer a theoretical framework that allows to initiate new lines of research focused on offering new methods and/or carefully analyzing the benefits, the methods of implementation and the evaluation of each one of the existing systems. About robotics, we have described how it has several benefits and alternatives; it has permitted human beings to have many different solutions to problems that one can find every day. Robotics has encouraged a lot of positive expectations in the medical field; as we have seen, there are many advantages such as speed, accuracy, precision and above everything else, more efficient work to improve our health and our iterations in it. With this technology, it has become possible to reach places of our anatomy that were very difficult to access in a way that gives specialists a higher success level in their work; the technology also offers the patient deeper confidence in accepting any type of intervention be it complex or very risky. IoMT is still learning from its experience, but it is going in the right direction and will be able to contribute to the existence of a social context in which there is no lack of security. It is mutually beneficial to have health and technology working together, because the workers of the medical service field are the main experts in the errors, failures, and violations that may exist in their devices. And the solution to these errors can only be offered by technology.

Chapter 3 titled, "An Overview on Wearable Devices for Medical Applications," is contributed by Meet Kumari and Meenu Gupta where they state that the whole word is facing Corona virus diseases. For this, social distancing is a major solution to overcome this disease, and wearable medical devices are the most attractive solution to help people. Wearable medical devices are the building block of modern healthcare systems having lots of stringent resource restrictions for providing lightweight healthcare facilities. This chapter provides an overview on the current significant research work done on wearable devices for medical applications. It categorizes the work according to the different types of wearable devices used for medical applications, the use of the wearable medical devices and different applications of wearable devices for medical applications. It also presents the various wearable medical devices parameters and their requirements in the current scenario. The potential open challenges faced by the current wearable medical devices and its future opportunities regarding its daily usage are also explained in this chapter. It is concluded that in spite of challenges, these wearable medical devices not only provide the numerous potential applications both socially and economically for real-time medical applications, but also they will be more helpful in hazardous working environments to provide safety in entire construction processes.

Chapter 4 titled, "Blockchain-Based IoT for Personalized Pharmaceuticals," is contributed by Rehab A. Rayan and Christos Tsagkaris. The chapter highlights the future healthcare system that will continue to have several electronic components. For example, using IoT could enable the housed data—both centrally, at the healthcare system level, or locally, at the patient level such as on a smartphone—to be critical components on selecting management approaches in a health-related condition. Producing medications and associated logistics is lagging far behind. For instance, cybersecurity and the needed strong public infrastructure are among the significant challenges. The cryptocurrency, a promising application of the blockchain technology, could revolutionize life sciences and biotechnology. The blockchain technique allows critical but lacking functionalities that are highly guarded and provide everlasting information housing, decentralizing and enhancing transaction transparency and incentivizing key stakeholders. A principal application of blockchain involves fighting fake medications with a focus on cryptopharmaceuticals technology, in which medications can be linked to a patient-specific blockchain of individual dosage units where every manufactured dosage unit has a distinctive information-rich model using a smartphone application to visualize such blockchain at all levels. These cover producing personalized dosage units and patients' views for their individual blockchain, and embedding such products into a healthy IoT system. Such a secured blockchain of individual medication history could avoid fake products and facilitates novel logistics. Hence, electronic ledgers could discover counterfeit drugs, facilitate virtual trials, and promote personalized medicine.

In Chapter 5, "Wearable/Implantable Devices for Monitoring Systems," contributed by Pawan Kumar and Shabana Urooj, the focus is on the use of antennas in various biomedical applications which is increasing day-by-day. The antennas are very useful in diagnosing and detecting various diseases without much hassle. A lot of research has been done on the design and use of the Wireless Capsule Endoscopy (WCE) which gives clear high-resolution images of the internal body organs (like the highly convoluted small intestine), which otherwise was a very difficult task using classic endoscopic techniques. Antennas have also played a key role in the treatment of diseases like cancer using hyperthermia, where the tumor cells can be targeted and burned. This enhances the effectiveness of other therapies like chemotherapy and radiotherapy which are being given to cancer patients.

Chapter 6, “Wearable Sensors for Monitoring Exercise and Fatigue Estimation in Rehabilitation,” is contributed by Maria J. Pinto-Bernal, Andres Aguirre, Carlos A. Cifuentes, and Marcela Munera. They stress that physical exercise has become a fundamental part of different rehabilitation environments. It is one of the main components of improving people’s health and decreasing morbidity and mortality levels through aerobic or anaerobic exercises. However, the intensity of these exercises must be controlled. Overtrained patients experiment with high states of fatigue that can affect their rehabilitation and health. In order to adjust these intensities, several methods have been explored to monitor the patients’ fatigue state to supervise exercise intensity during therapies. Nevertheless, these methods often need to be adapted to the environment and the patients, making their implementation difficult. In this context, this chapter presents the importance of physical exercise in rehabilitation, traditional fatigue monitoring strategies, and strategies for monitoring based on wearable sensors with massive potential for estimating fatigue levels. Finally, this chapter presents two experimental studies to estimate performance-related fatigue in an aerobic and anaerobic exercise using wearable sensors. The preliminary results show that the use of wearable sensors would measure and indicate the fatigue reflected in spatial-temporal parameters and kinematic parameters during the execution of aerobic and anaerobic exercises.

Chapter 7 is titled, “Conversational Agents for Healthcare Delivery: Potential Solutions to the Challenges of the Pandemic,” and is submitted by Laura M. Bautista, Marcela Munera, and Carlos A. Cifuentes. In this chapter, the authors talk about the Conversational Agents (CAs) for healthcare delivery which have been emerging rapidly due to their potential to improve the quality of life of the patients and the level of healthcare and reduce costs. As CAs evolved, so did wearable devices, advances such as heart rate monitors, smartwatches, activity monitors, and other wearable sensors, have made mobile devices ideal units for healthcare delivery that, working together with CAs, open up a new and growing world of opportunities. The possibility of innovation through the use of wearable devices with the intervention of CAs could allow in some cases immediate feedback, supplementing the shortage of staff in primary healthcare centers thereby reducing the burden on service providers. In this chapter, the authors present a review of existing systems that use wearable devices in joint work with a conversational agent to create a new way of healthcare delivery through an interactive personalized service that can be carried out in both hospital and home conditions. The results of the first experiments and pilot studies of these systems have demonstrated their acceptance and effectiveness.

Chapter 8 titled, “Role of Big Data in e-Healthcare Application for Managing a Large Amount of Data,” is contributed by Meenu Gupta, Dr. Rachna Jain, Rachit Singhal and Jaspreet Singh. It discusses the medical researchers’ work with huge amounts of data for managing their treatment plans and analyzing recovery rates of their patients. To examine tumor samples, biobanks linked up with their patient treatment records which may consist of a large amount of data. In old times, we were working on much less data. As time passes, every day data grows. To manage this data was a critical issue for industries (or companies). This data can be defined in any form such as a phone log book, email or any other sources. Collecting data is very easy, but to manage it is very difficult. Then, cloud computing came into the picture to store huge amounts of data on a server. But, every day we are generating data in gigabytes, which is very difficult to manage. Big Data advances and reduces this storage problem of data on a server. Big Data provides a framework called "Hadoop" which helps to store a large amount of data on a server. Managing data at a large scale was the motivation behind writing this chapter. This chapter discusses the technologies used in Hadoop and how they are beneficial for medical healthcare system. The principal aim of this chapter is to make people familiar with the role of Big Data Hadoop and how to deal with a large amount of data. Many mobile applications or biometric sensors generate a large amount of data related to healthcare. It is very important to understand generated data and overcome issues of this generated data by different health monitoring applications. In this chapter the most used technologies are discussed for handling Big Data starting from the old-school methods of manual analysis and moving on to advanced technologies like Spark, Kafka, etc. Some of these technologies like manual analysis and MRP systems have been replaced by new technologies. However, a plethora of technologies still exist in the market. As a result, organizations dealing with Big Data have to choose the right technology to use for handling Big Data related to the healthcare industry. The main questions that arise while choosing the correct platform is what the requirements of the organization are and what outcome they expect if they deploy a certain scheme. In addition, managers have to take cost and storage factors into account as well. Selecting the right platform is tough as well as a complicated step. Furthermore, once an organization commits, then adopting something different is difficult as well as expensive. Every major company and organization is using Big Data nowadays to organize large amounts of health-related data. The use of Big Data has grown to encompass multiple industries and fields. Big Data facilitates healthcare in terms of predicting health-related issues. After analysis of Big Data, EHRs, EMRs and other medical data is continuously helping build a better prognostic framework. The companies providing service for healthcare analytics and clinical transformation are indeed contributing towards a better and effective outcome.

Editors

Dr. Manuel Cardona, Ph.D. received the B.S. degree in Electrical Engineering in El Salvador, in 2004 and the Master degree in Automation and Robotics from Universidad Politécnica de Madrid, Spain, in 2008. From 2007 to 2008, and 2011, he was a research assistant with the Robotics and Intelligence Machines Research Group at Universidad Politécnica de Madrid, Spain. He has a Postgraduate Degree in Scientific Research and a Postgraduate Degree and Innovation Management. In 2020, he received the Ph.D. (Cum Laude) in Automation and Robotics from Universidad Politécnica de Madrid, Spain. Currently, he is the research director and the director of the Robotics and Intelligence Machines Research Group and Computer Vision Research Group at Universidad Don Bosco (UDB), El Salvador. His research interest includes rehabilitation robotics, biomechanics, kinematic and dynamic of serial and parallel robots, embedded systems, vision and artificial intelligence, and applications of robotics systems. He has authored or co-authored more than 45 research articles that are published in various journals, books, and conference proceedings. He is an associate editor of *International Journal of Machine Learning and Networked Collaborative Engineering (IJMLNCE)*, ISSN 2581-3242. He is an IEEE senior member and belongs to Robotics and Automation Society (RAS), Aerospace and Electronic Systems Society (AESS), and Education Society (EdSOC). He is IEEE RAS and AESS student branch chapter advisor and student branch mentor at Universidad Don Bosco, and the vice chair at IEEE, El Salvador Section.

Vijender Kumar Solanki, Ph.D., is an associate professor in Computer Science & Engineering, CMR Institute of Technology (Autonomous), Hyderabad, TS, India. He has more than 10 years of academic experience in network security, IoT, Big Data, Smart City and IT. Prior to his current role, he was associated with Apeejay Institute of Technology, Greater Noida, UP, KSRCE (Autonomous) Institution, Tamilnadu, India and Institute of Technology & Science, Ghaziabad, UP, India. He is a member of ACM and IEEE.

He has attended an orientation program at UGC-Academic Staff College, University of Kerala, Thiruvananthapuram, Kerala and took a refresher course at the Indian Institute of Information Technology, Allahabad, UP, India.

He has authored or co-authored more than 50 research articles that are published in various journals, books and conference proceedings. He has edited or co-edited 14 books and conference proceedings in the area of Soft Computing.

He received a Ph.D. in Computer Science and Engineering from Anna University, Chennai, India in 2017 and an ME, MCA from Maharishi Dayanand University, Rohtak, Haryana, India in 2007 and 2004, respectively, and a B.S from JLN Government College, Faridabad Haryana, India in 2001.

He is the book series editor of the following: *Internet of Everything (IoE): Security and Privacy Paradigm*, CRC Press, Taylor & Francis Group, USA; *Artificial Intelligence (AI): Elementary to Advanced Practices Series*, CRC Press,

Taylor & Francis Group, USA; *IT, Management & Operations Research Practices*, CRC Press, Taylor & Francis Group, USA; *Bio-Medical Engineering: Techniques and Applications*, Apple Academic Press, USA; and *Computational Intelligence and Management Science Paradigm, (Focus Series)*, CRC Press, Taylor & Francis Group, USA.

He is editor-in-chief of the *International Journal of Machine Learning and Networked Collaborative Engineering (IJMLNCE)*, ISSN 2581-3242; *International Journal of Hyperconnectivity and the Internet of Things (IJHIoT)*, IGI-Global, USA, ISSN 2473-4365. He is also co-editor of *Ingenieria Solidaria Journal*, ISSN (2357-6014); associate editor of the *International Journal of Information Retrieval Research (IJIRR)*, IGI-Global, USA, ISSN: 2155-6377|E-ISSN: 2155-6385. He has been guest editor with IGI-Global, USA, InderScience and many more publishers. He can be contacted at: spesinfo@yahoo.com or vijendersolanki@ieee.org

Cecilia E. García Cena, Ph.D., received her B.S. degree in Electromechanics Engineering from La Pampa National University, Santa Rosa, Argentina, in 1997 and a Ph.D. degree in Control Systems (curriculum in robotics and nonlinear system control) from San Juan National University, San Juan, Argentina, in 2001.

In 2001, she was a visiting scholar with the Robotics Section, Universidad Politécnica de Madrid (UPM-CSIC), Madrid, Spain. In 2004, she was a visiting professor with the Robotics Laboratory, Universidad Carlos III de Madrid, Madrid.

She is currently a professor with the Department of Electronics, Automation and Computer Science, UPM-CSIC, and a member of the Centre of Automation and Robotics, UPM-CSIC. Her research interests include telerobotics, assistant robots, and control of multiagent systems. She holds three patents and is the author of more than 20 articles.

Contributors

Andres Aguirre
Department of Biomedical Engineering
Colombian School of Engineering Julio Garavito
Bogotá, Colombia

Margarita Bautista
Department of Biomedical Engineering
Colombian School of Engineering Julio Garavito
Bogotá, Colombia

Lucia Alonso Virgos
Universidad International de la Rioja (UNIR)
Logroño, Spain

Maria J. Pinto-Bernal
Department of Biomedical Engineering
Colombian School of Engineering Julio Garavito
Bogotá, Colombia

Claudia L. Garzón-Castro
Facultad de Ingeniería
Universidad de La Sabana
Campus Universitario del Puente del Común
Chía, Cundinamarca, Colombia

Carlos A. Cifuentes
Department of Biomedical Engineering
Colombian School of Engineering Julio Garavito
Bogotá, Colombia

J. Javier Rainer Granados
Universidad International de la Rioja (UNIR)
Logroño, Spain

Meenu Gupta
Department of Computer Science and Engineering
Chandigarh University
Chandigarh, India

Fernando López Hernández
Universidad International de la Rioja (UNIR)
Logroño, Spain

Rachna Jain
Department of Computer Science and Engineering
Bharati Vidyapeeth's College of Engineering
Delhi, India

Pawan Kumar
Department of Electrical Engineering
School of Engineering, Gautam Buddha University
Greater Noida, India

Meet Kumari
Department of Electronics and Communication Engineering
Chandigarh University
Chandigarh, India

Marcela Munera
Department of Biomedical Engineering
Colombian School of Engineering Julio Garavito
Bogotá, Colombia

Rehab A. Rayan
Department of Epidemiology
High Institute of Public Health
Alexandria University
Alexandria, Egypt

Jaspreet Singh
Department of Computer Science and Engineering
Chandigarh University
Chandigarh, India

Rachit Singhal
Department of Computer Science and Engineering
Bharati Vidyapeeth's College of Engineering
Delhi, India

Christos Tsagkaris
Faculty of Medicine
University of Crete
Heraklion, Greece

Ramiro Velázquez
Facultad de Ingeniería
Universidad Panamericana
Aguascalientes, México

Miguel A. Sanchez Vidales
Universidad International de la Rioja (UNIR)
Logroño, Spain

Shabana Urooj
Department of Electrical Engineering
School of Engineering, Gautam Buddha University
Greater Noida, India

1 Fundamentals and Paradigms in the Internet of Things

Claudia Lorena Garzón-Castro[1]
and Ramiro Velázquez[2]
[1]Universidad de La Sabana, Facultad de Ingeniería, Campus Universitario del Puente del Común, Km 7 Autopista Norte de Bogotá, Chía, Cundinamarca, Colombia.
[2]Universidad Panamericana, Facultad de Ingeniería, Josemaría Escrivá de Balaguer 101, Fracc. Rústicos Calpulli, C.P. 20290, Aguascalientes, México.

CONTENTS

1.1 Introduction 1
1.2 IoT Characteristics 2
1.3 Architectures for IoT 3
1.4 Sensors, Actuators, and Data Storage 7
1.5 Communication Protocols 8
1.6 User Interface Properties 8
1.7 IoT in Healthcare: Benefits, Developments, and Challenges 9
1.7.1 Benefits 9
1.7.2 Examples of IoT-Based Healthcare Devices 10
1.7.3 Challenges 14
1.8 Conclusions 14
References 15

1.1 INTRODUCTION

The term Internet of Things (IoT) was first used in 1999 by the British technology pioneer Kevin Ashton, who worked at Procter & Gamble (P&G) [1]. This new paradigm emerged as the solution to the lack of information P&G had in order to determine when and where its most popular products sold out in stores. The solution proposed by Ashton was to include sensors in their products so they would be able track and count everything in order to greatly reduce waste, losses and overall costs. This way, they would be able to know when a product was out of stock [2]. However, it was not until 2009 that this paradigm took off, turning into the third revolutionary wave in computing technology after the personal computer and Internet [3]. This was accomplished because the IoT has the capability to collect, analyze and dispense data that we can transform into information and knowledge [4].

In the literature, there are many definitions for the Internet of Things also known as the Internet of Objects [5–10] or Web 3.0 [11]. In general, it can be said that the IoT aims for a world where everything, including houses, home appliances, cars, urban furniture and industrial machinery are connected to the Internet at any given time and place, creating real-time data that facilitates decision making, offering the user comfort while saving time and money.

Because of the attributes that IoT has, in 2008, the US National Intelligence Council (NIC) included the IoT in the list of six "Disruptive Civil Technologies" with potential impacts on US national power. In their report, the NIC said that by 2025, everyday objects like food containers could be nodes on the Internet. Furthermore, the NIC highlighted that the IoT could play a key role in the economic development and the military capacity of the United States of America. However, the NIC also mentioned that there will be information security risks when people gain the ability to control, locate and monitor their devices remotely [12].

The emergence of the IoT is an evolutionary result of a series of existing technologies like wireless sensor networks (WSNs), actuators, network communication means and protocols [13, 14], storage and computing tools for data analysis and visualization and interpretation tools which can be widely accessed on different platforms [11]. The IoT sets a significative interaction between people, machines and smart devices contributing to the quality of life, helping people make decisions and grow the world economy [13, 15]. In addition, the IoT is characterized by helping to reduce the carbon footprint. Without a doubt, the paradigm has made a significant impact from the labor to the domestic field. This has allowed the range of IoT applications to include a wide spectrum of real-world applications as healthcare, agriculture, process management, mass production, environmental and urban infrastructure control, intelligent transportation and logistics systems, the energy industry, and security and surveillance, among others [7, 14–17]. Of all these fields of action, it should be noted that the IoT is really making a difference in the healthcare sector.

This chapter aims to present the fundamentals of the IoT. The rest of the chapter is organized as follows: Section 1.2 addresses the most relevant characteristics of the IoT. Section 1.3 overviews the layers of the three most popular architectures in IoT. In Section 1.4, the sensors, actuators, and storage used in IoT-based applications are described. The most commonly used communication protocols for the IoT are given in Section 1.5. Section 1.6 points to the characteristics that should be taken into account for the development of user interfaces. Section 1.7 presents the benefits, some application examples, and challenges of the IoT in the healthcare industry. Finally, the conclusions are given in Section 1.8.

1.2 IoT CHARACTERISTICS

Regardless of the application and associated technology used for the implementation of the IoT, the type of architecture must have some fundamental characteristics that allow it to provide a good service to end users. Some of the characteristics that identify the IoT are:

- Things: Also known as objects or devices. These are the main actors of the IoT. These are made to make users' lives more comfortable. These devices must have communication and detection/actuation capabilities [18]. Therefore, they are equipped with sensors and actuators. The detection/actuation capacity is important, especially with those that represent the interface with the user and the coupling between the physical and the virtual world [19].
- Connectivity: This feature should enable communication, integration and assignment of a single address to the IoT devices. In the IoT, there is currently a wide range of connectivity options, which will surely adapt in order to meet the demands of emerging IoT devices [19].
- Data: The data obtained from the interconnection between devices is the IoT's value. This value is enhanced by the intelligent analysis and use of the collected data [19].
- Autonomy: This feature allows IoT-based devices to carry out their tasks without the intervention of humans or any other devices [20].
- Services: These must be available to interact with IoT devices, taking into account restrictions such as privacy protection and semantic consistency between IoT devices and virtual objects [18].
- Heterogeneity: Given the diversity of IoT devices, the design is required of appropriate solutions that allow their integration through communication protocols, inferior technologies and access to resources within the interconnection solution that is available. [19].
- Security: This feature is extremely important for the benefits of the IoT to remain useful. Therefore, endpoints, networks and data must be secured [21].
- Autoconfiguration (plug and play): This feature seeks that IoT devices can support their configuration automatically [20].

1.3 ARCHITECTURES FOR IoT

The IoT architecture must ensure that data are transported, stored, processed and made available to the user [22]. Thus, the search for an IoT architecture that supports the different environments and contexts of the world has been a challenge. Hence, it is important to have a modular and scalable architecture that allows the integration of new functionalities. In the literature, there are a number of proposed architectures which are typically divided into levels. The three best known architectures are as follows:

1. **Three-layer architecture:** This architecture contemplates the perception layer, network layer and application layer [8, 23], see Figure 1.1. Next, a description is made of the most important characteristics of each of these layers.

   The perception layer: This layer is also known as the terminal layer or the device layer. The perception layer is classified in two sections: the perception node (sensors, actuators, etc.) and the perception network that is responsible for interconnecting the network layer. Data are acquired and controlled at the perception node [24]. The main task of this level is to

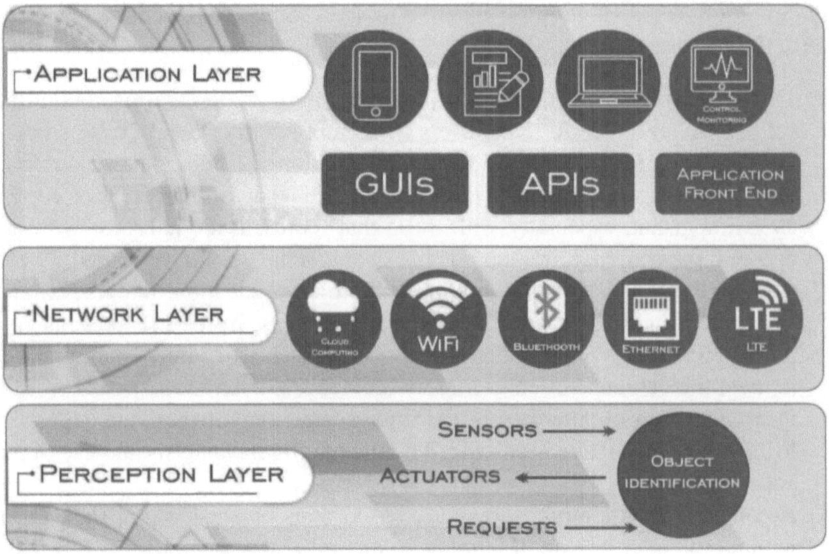

FIGURE 1.1 Three-layer architecture schematic for IoT.

identify the object by collecting information through the use of sensors. This information is transmitted over the network as digital signals. This level may also include code labels and readers, Radio Frequency Identification (RFID), video cameras, sensors, Wireless Sensor Networks (WSNs), and others.

The network layer: Also known as the transport layer. The main function of this layer is transmitting and processing the data coming from the perception layer; in other words, it supports the connectivity of the devices. Data transmission between networks can be achieved using wired and wireless communications. This is why the network layer is made up of all those technologies with which one can access the Internet, such as: 3G, 4G, Wi-Fi, Long-Term Evolution (LTE), ZigBee, and Bluetooth, among others. This layer may have different communication protocols, since it must ensure communication between different networks. Some of the protocols used are: IPV6 (6LoWPAN), Message Queue Telemetry Transport (MQTT), Constrained Application Protocol (CoAP), HTTP, DDS, and AMQP.

The application layer: At this level, various types of developments and user services can be found, which make use of the data collected at the perception level. Furthermore, this layer allows data to be shared with other applications and platforms [16] through Application Programming Interfaces (APIs) or Graphical User Interfaces (GUIs) [22]. The application layer encompasses the most functional modules in the IoT system. This layer assists as the front-end interface to offer analysis and decision-making results for users. The various applications can be grouped in three main domains: the industrial domain, e.g., transportation and logistics; the health welfare domain, e.g., health care; and the smart city domain [25]. Some of the technologies used are augmented intelligence and augmented cognition.

The application layer in this three-layer architecture corresponds to the services and applications layers in the four-layer architecture, or the business, applications and middleware layers in the five-layer architecture [15].

2. **Four-layer architecture:** This architecture is service-oriented, which corresponds to the middleware layer of the five-layer architecture [26]. The services layer, also known as the processing layer, is in charge of storing the data delivered by the network layer, analyzing valuable information and making decisions. This layer is capable of managing and providing a series of services to the lower layers. A diagram of this architecture is shown in Figure 1.2. The main characteristics of the functions of this layer are [27]:

Data validation: This action is performed to verify the integrity of the source.

Data transformation: In order to store the data, it must be transformed into several or into a single format. However, given the different applications, regardless of the format in which the storage was performed, the data may require an additional format change.

Data filtering: Corresponds to the separation of the data according to the utility in the developed application.

Data processing and storage: This function is given by the amount of data that can be generated, so it is recommended to use Big Data technology to obtain useful information.

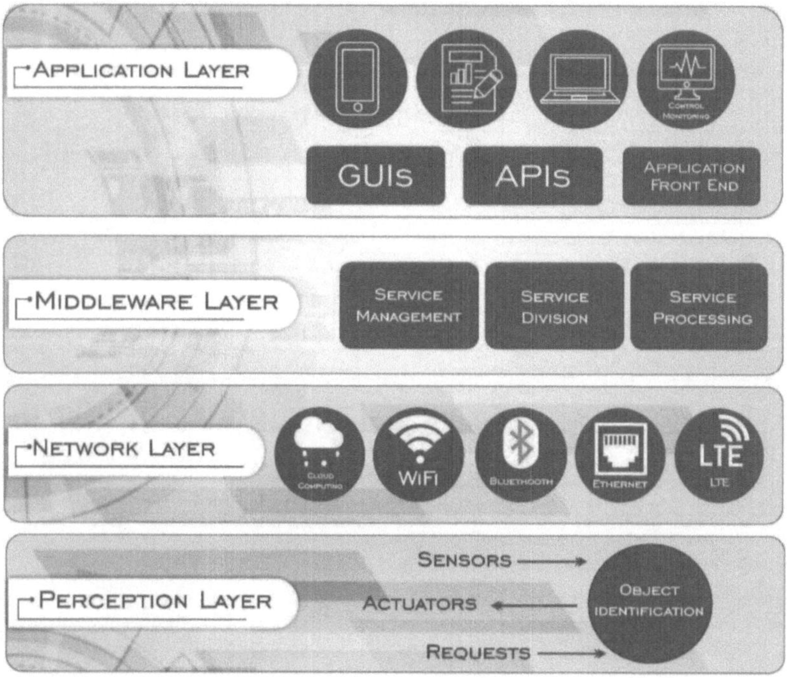

FIGURE 1.2 Four-layer architecture schematic for IoT.

Registry of entities: The different elements, such as users, devices and services, must be identified and registered as entities of the system so that it is possible to have a registry of entities, establish relationships and make associations between them.

Protocol support: To guarantee a good service, it is necessary to guarantee communication with heterogeneous networks, support various gateways and devices, and integrate new protocols.

3. **Five-layer architecture:** In this case, the business layer is added. The responsibilities of this layer are to manage the applications, build the business model, generate the charts and flow charts, etc. The above is based on data from the application layer [23, 28]. The business layer supports decision making by doing a Big Data analysis [15]. Additionally, it must also manage the security of the IoT system, where functions such as: authentication, user privacy, and authorizations, among others, must be provided [16]. Finally, this layer is also responsible for monitoring and managing the lower layers. Figure 1.3 shows this architecture.

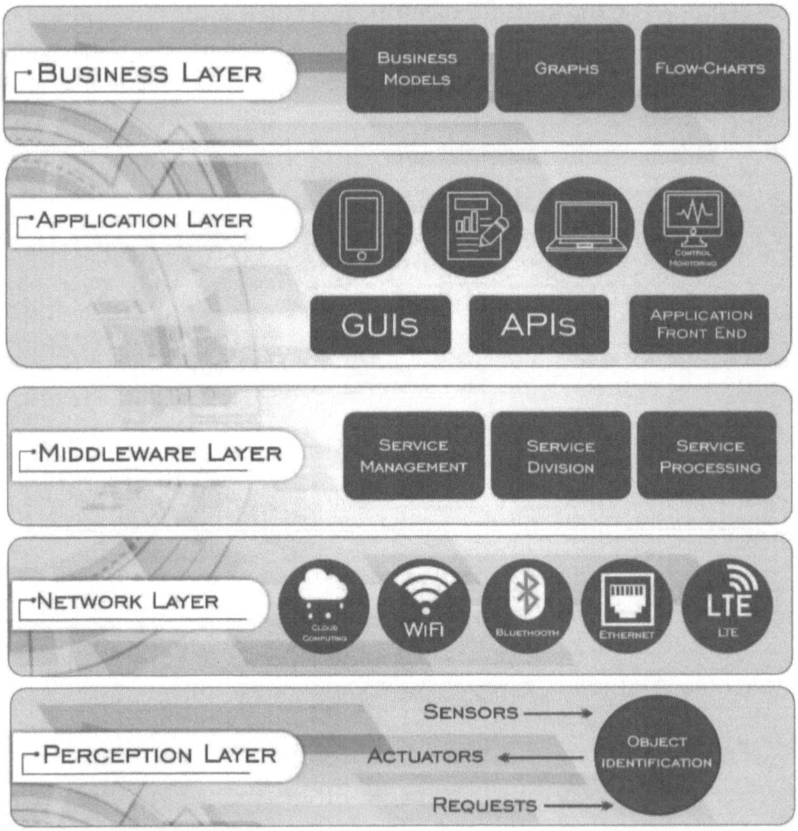

FIGURE 1.3 Five-layer architecture schematic for IoT.

TABLE 1.1
Sensor Classification According to the IoT Application

Category	Examples
Ambient sensors	Temperature, light, atmospheric pressure, humidity sensors
Motion sensors	Accelerometers, gyroscopes
Electric sensors	Current, tension, capacitive sensors
Biosensors	Electrocardiogram (ECG), electroencephalogram (EEG), heartbeat, breath sensors
Object identification	Smart tags, beacons
Position sensors	GPS, magnetometers, fixed wireless access points
Presence sensors	Passive infrared sensor (PIR), video cameras
Interaction sensors	Physical buttons, tactile tablets, sliders
Acoustic sensors	Microphones
Environmental sensors	Smoke detectors, pH, gas sensors

1.4 SENSORS, ACTUATORS, AND DATA STORAGE

IoT sensors are regular sensors with the slight difference that their output signals are connected to the network. A recent survey of the literature on IoT-based applications [29] classifies the sensors as summarized in Table 1.1.

On the other hand, IoT actuators are regular actuators with the difference that their input signals come from the network. Table 1.2 summarizes the type of actuators commonly found in IoT-based applications.

One of the key characteristics of the IoT architecture is that the cloud server centralizes all data collected from the set of sensors. Therefore, it is the module responsible for data storage.

There are several major cloud storage providers such as Microsoft Azure, Amazon Web Services (AWS), and Google Cloud.

Cloud storage offers the following advantages:

1. **Equipment cost reduction:** Cloud storage allows cutting expenses related to hardware such as servers and hard drives.

TABLE 1.2
Actuator Classification According to the IoT Application

Category	Role in the IoT Environment
Linear actuators	Used to enable object motion in a straight line
Motors	Used to rotate mechanisms or objects with high positioning accuracy
Relays	Electromagnet actuators used to power devices
Solenoids	Widely used in home appliances (locking/triggering mechanisms and monitoring systems)

2. **Staff cost reduction:** Cloud storage offers a non-stop service. Cloud servers and data centers are managed by the cloud service provided. Therefore, there is no need for IT employee management.
3. **Cloud storage is scalable and reliable:** Data is safely stored in the cloud and storage capacity can be customized. Most cloud providers have data centers in various locations around the world, which allows a faster data processing and a more reliable storage.

1.5 COMMUNICATION PROTOCOLS

Communication protocols are considered the backbone of IoT-based systems, as they enable network connectivity and data exchange over the network. They determine data encoding, data exchange formats, and package routing from source to destination. They are also involved in sequence control, flow control, and retransmission of lost packets [30].

The following protocols are the most commonly used in IoT:

1. **IEEE 802.11 – WiFi:** WiFi is a collection of Wireless Local Area Network (WLAN) communication standards: 802.11a, 802.11b, 802.11ac, and 802.11ad operating in the band range of 2.4 to 60 GHz. They provide data exchange rates from 1 Mb/s to 6.75 Gb/s and a communication range in the order of 20 m (indoor) to 100 m (outdoor).
2. **IEEE 802.16 – WiMAX:** WiMAX (Worldwide Interoperability for Microwave Access) provides data exchange rates from 1.5 Mb/s to 1 Gb/s. It provides an average data rate of 100 Mb/s for mobile stations and 1 Gb/s for fixed stations.
3. **IEEE 802.15.1 – Bluetooth:** Bluetooth is a low-power, low-cost wireless communication technology suitable for data transmission between mobile devices over a short range (8–10 m). It operates in the 2.4 GHz band.
4. **LoRaWAN – LoRa:** LoRaWAN is a newly developed long-range communication protocol. Its aim is to guarantee interoperability between various operators in one open global standard. LoRaWAN data exchange rates range from 0.3 kb/s to 50 kb/s. LoRa operates in 868 and 900 MHz bands. LoRa is capable of communicating nodes located 30 km apart.

1.6 USER INTERFACE PROPERTIES

As it was previously stated, the IoT can be successfully used to manage services in systems of diverse areas, including functions such as: signal monitoring, remote device activation, problem detection, service management, and access to reports, among others. These functions must be available to the user in an application (App) through a User Interface (UI). This UI must allow the user to interact with the information and the device on which the App is hosted. According to [31], if the UI is well designed, the user will be able to view and receive the information quickly and intuitively; otherwise, the user will be frustrated. The most used UIs for the development of these Apps are the Graphical User Interfaces (GUIs).

According to the experts, there is no adequate design for all user groups, which makes the development of applications important based on the characteristics of the target group [32]. Therefore, one can find studies focused on taking into account certain psychological factors of users when developing GUIs [33]. For example, in [31] they designed an assistive App for children with autism with the use of a touch-screen. The objective of this App is to help children learn, memorize and recognize numbers and thus be able to perform basic mathematical calculations. While in [34] the development of an intuitive GUI to handle the Brain–Computer Interface (BCI) system, looking to reach high classification and Information Transfer Rates (ITRs) is presented. Finally, in [35] the authors developed an investigation of the characteristics that a UI should have, which would allow older people suffering from dementia to have an intuitive interaction with the performance of Activities of Daily Living (ADLs), such as, for example, the handling of a microwave oven. In this case, the researchers found that for older people with dementia, simple designs were optimal.

In short, according to [32], some of the principles that should be taken into account when designing UIs are: (a) reduce the amount of available functions, i.e., reduce the complexity of the software, (b) design an interface that allows to easily find tools, (c) use larger icons to show key software functions, (d) avoid using technical terms, (e) customize font, font color and size, and (f) use graphic objects like avatars or icons.

Finally, another feature to consider when developing an App is the type of access that should be given to each user. This feature gives a different view to data analytics according to the privileges given to the user. In these cases, when the user logs in, a service is run to obtain the user privileges and user interface components that they will be able to see. This type of App is known as a cross-platform application [36]. In some cases, the user will be able to access and edit the information, while in other cases the user will only have permission to consult the data.

1.7 IoT IN HEALTHCARE: BENEFITS, DEVELOPMENTS, AND CHALLENGES

The IoT has undoubtedly affected the healthcare industry. Its incorporation has brought benefits that have improved the efficiency and quality of therapies, treatments, and follow- ups that have positively impacted the health and lives of patients.

1.7.1 Benefits

Among the palpable benefits of the IoT in healthcare we can identify:

1. **Remote medical assistance:** IoT solutions allow physicians to assist patients who can be located remotely. Physicians can talk to the patients, check their vital signals using specialized Apps and Internet-connected monitoring devices, diagnose them, and prescribe the corresponding medicines. Besides the benefits to the patient, remote medical assistance impacts hospital costs as well: IoT is moving medical appointments from hospitals (hospital-centric) to the patients' homes (home-centric) optimizing infrastructure resources.

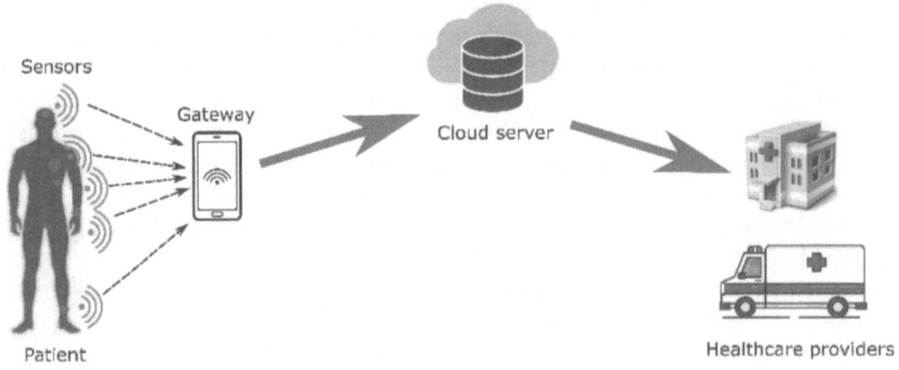

FIGURE 1.4 The general architecture of an IoT-based healthcare system.

2. **Instantaneous tracking and alerts:** Real-time pertinent alerts are of extreme value in life-threatening events. IoT healthcare devices are capable of collecting vital data and transferring them to physicians and emergency services for a prompt reaction.
3. **Automated reporting:** Raw data obtained from patients needs to be further processed in order to arrive to a clinical conclusion. Healthcare providers devote a significant amount of time in manually collecting, reporting, and analyzing such raw data. The IoT has the capacity of automating these processes even with a vast amount of data coming from several monitoring devices; thus allowing physicians, hospitals, and healthcare organizations to speed up diagnosis.
4. **Ease of healthcare research:** The IoT has become a valuable tool for healthcare research purposes. The massive amount of data it offers accelerates the statistical study of diseases and medical conditions that would eventually enable the implementation of better therapies and treatments.

The schematic in Figure 1.4 shows the general architecture of an IoT-based service in healthcare. A number of sensors monitor in real time diverse physiological signals. Among the most popular sensors we can find are electroencephalogram (EEG) sensors, electrocardiogram (ECG) sensors, respiratory rate sensors, pulse sensors, and motion sensors. Using a gateway, data are uploaded and centralized in a cloud server to be later analyzed by healthcare professionals. The gateway is the device that provides the bridge between the sensors and the cloud. The most commonly used device nowadays is the smartphone.

1.7.2 Examples of IoT-Based Healthcare Devices

This subsection aims to present some representative examples of IoT-based devices devoted to healthcare.

Villalpando et al. presented in [37] a medical briefcase conceived to be used as a telemedicine system. The medical briefcase is a set of computer-based medical

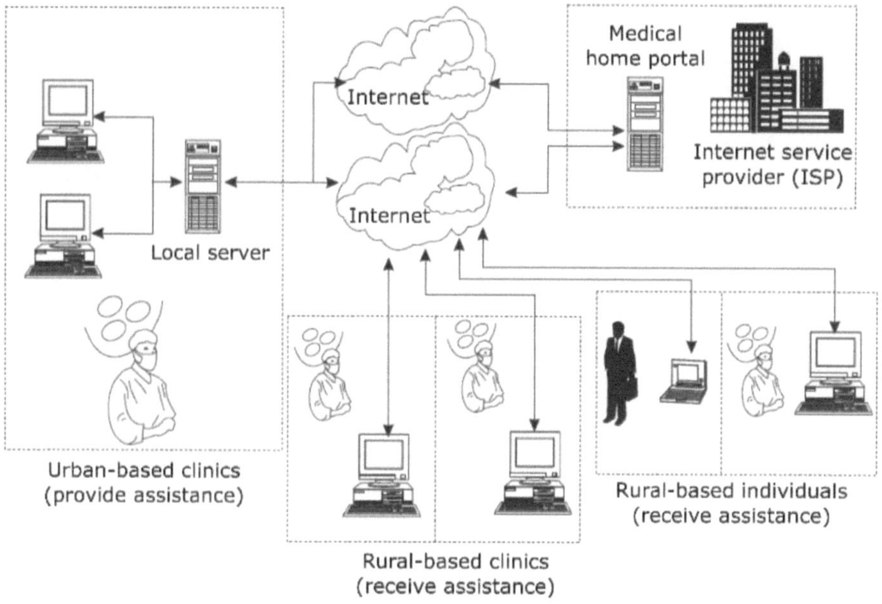

FIGURE 1.5 The medical briefcase architecture: Interaction of specialized physicians, rural-based physicians, and rural-based patients using an IoT telediagnosis scheme.

instrumentation that offers not only the basic characteristics of traditional medical instrumentation, but also the capability of analysis and remote transmission of physiological information in order to perform telediagnosis tasks. One of its main advantages is that it encompasses advanced digital signal processing algorithms [38] that offer high quality results in cardiology diagnosis and telediagnosis at low cost. It is devoted to reach patients located in rural areas in Mexico.

The medical briefcase encompasses an ECG, a Holter (ambulatory ECG), a pulse oximeter, a digital stethoscope, a digital thermometer, and a baumanometer (blood pressure meter). Its architecture is shown in Figure 1.5.

The medical briefcase enables medical assistance to patients, physicians, and clinics based in rural communities or remote locations. Collected data in these locations are uploaded to a cloud server-based medical portal, which is ensured by an Internet provider. Data is to be analyzed by specialists based on a central clinic or hospital located in cities. The idea is to assist rural physicians with specialized diagnosis without the barriers of distance.

A number of systems for telemonitoring of physiological signals have been developed and can be found in the literature: heart signals [39, 40], brain signals [41, 42], respiratory activity [43, 44], and blood parameters [45, 46], among others. All of them are devoted to perform a real-time follow-up of the patient health status to ensure a prompt medical response.

Jian and Chen introduced in [47] a portable fall detection and alerting system for remote monitoring and timely assistance of elderly people. Such system basically consists of a custom vest and a mobile smartphone. The vest integrates a motion

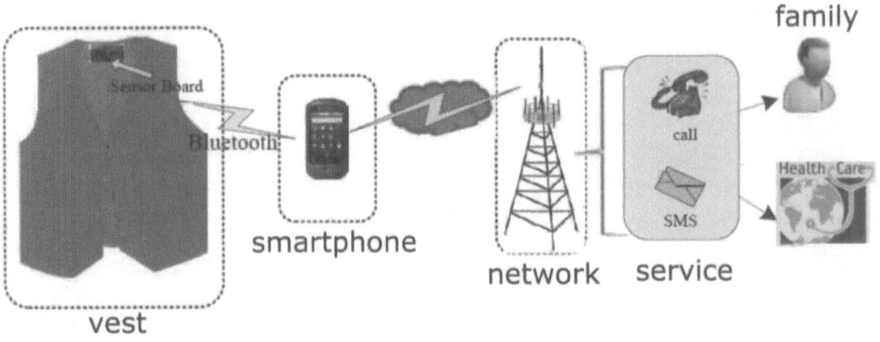

FIGURE 1.6 IoT-based wearable system for fall detection.

detection sensor with a tri-axial accelerometer and gyroscope. When the sensor detects abrupt changes of acceleration and velocity, data is sent to a smartphone via Bluetooth. An alert is sent to a family member or a healthcare center to provide timely assistance. The architecture of this system is shown in Figure 1.6.

Similar IoT-based alert systems have been proposed for a wide number of applications. Kattukkaran et al. described in [48] an accident detection and alert system consisting of an accelerometer placed on the vehicle and a heartbeat sensor. Both sensors are connected to a mobile phone via Bluetooth. When an abnormality is detected, the mobile phone sends an alert to the nearest medical center providing the GPS coordinates of the accident. Pawlak and coworkers proposed in [49] the Medical Cyber-Physical System (MCPS) an IoT-based system for telemonitoring pregnant women at home. The MCPS monitors abdominal signals and provides alerts of eventualities to a central surveillance center located in a hospital. To monitor the continuous and timely usage of medicines by elderly people, Kuwik et al. implemented a smart medical dispenser [50]. Such dispenser tracks the use of prescribed medicine by patients and alerts physicians, healthcare providers, or family members if the patient does not access the medicine in a set time frame.

IoT in healthcare is not just about capturing physiological signals, processing them, and sending SOS alerts. This technology can also be used in Assistive Technologies (AT) and rehabilitation.

Velázquez et al. [51] reported an AT wearable device devoted to assist blind and visually impaired users while navigating outdoors. Urban navigation is a major challenge for visually disabled people, as they have to find their way along the environment together with constant obstacle detection [52]. This system targets to assist users in finding their destinations. For this purpose, the concept in Figure 1.7 was proposed. The system consists of a smartphone and an on-shoe tactile display.

Figure 1.8 shows its operation principle. Using the smartphone's Internet connectivity, the user's geospatial information is transmitted to a cloud server. The smartphone updates the server at 5 Hz, which extensively covers any walking speed. A remote computer accesses the server's information and locates the user in a locally running spatial database. The Geographic Information System (GIS) used in this project is OpenStreetMap [53]. A dedicated script links to the YOURS Application

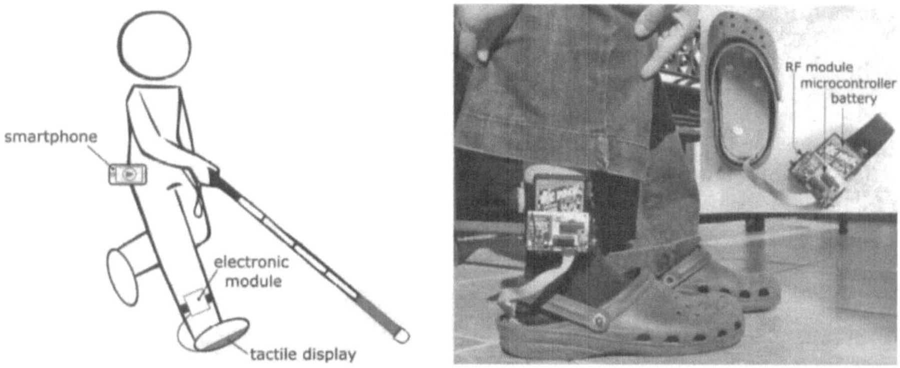

FIGURE 1.7 Concept and prototype of a wearable navigation assistive device for blind people.

Programming Interface (API) [54], an open-source route planner, to compute the shortest pedestrian route to a previously chosen destination. The route waypoints are returned from YOURS, and they are placed and stored in the GIS. Directions to the destination are processed locally. Directions are translated to actuator commands, which are transmitted via radiofrequency (RF) to an electronic module that the user carries with him/her. Finally, signals are interpreted by a microcontroller, which sets the actuators in the tactile display.

Hence, users perceive directions encoded as vibrations. A comprehensive study on tactile-foot perception [55] has shown that this information is easy to understand and that it actually has the potential to point directions to blind people.

Several IoT devices for AT and rehabilitation have been proposed. Su et al. introduced in [56] a set of customized home-based games for muscle and working

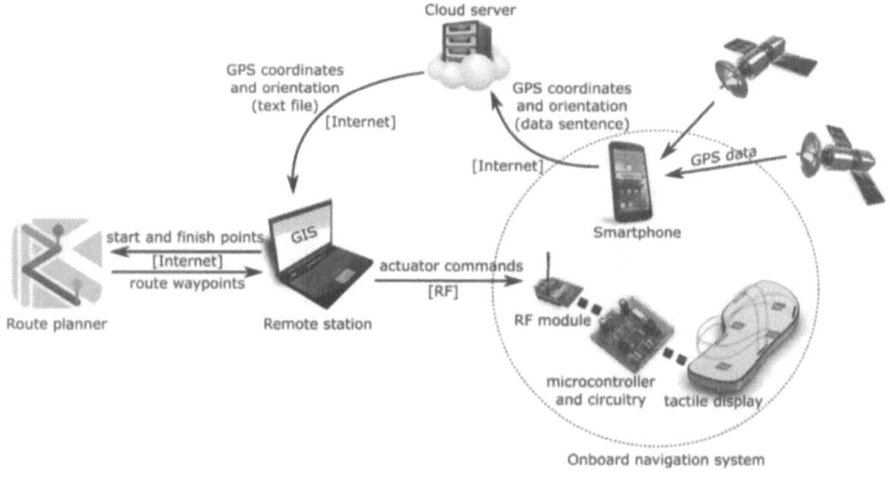

FIGURE 1.8 IoT-based operation principle of the AT device.

memory training. Devoted to prevent functional deterioration of the elderly, results are monitored remotely. Yang and colleagues reported in [57] a rehabilitation system for upper-limb stroke patients connected to the cloud that is capable of collecting data on a daily basis to perform a close tracking of their rehabilitation progress. A last example is the work developed by Sula et al. [58] in which an IoT-based system for supporting learning and improving the quality of life for children with Autism Spectrum Disorder (ASD) was presented.

1.7.3 Challenges

Even though IoT-based technology offers a wide number of advantages, it also poses several challenges. Among them, it is possible to identify:

1. **Data security and patient privacy:** IoT devices collect and transmit sensitive data both synchronously and asynchronously. Data is stored in the cloud and then accessed from different locations. There are undoubtedly too many access points where security could be compromised. In addition, nowadays there is significant ambiguity regarding data ownership over time and regulations are still to be designed.
2. **Multiple protocols:** IoT devices are based on a number of different protocols such as Wi-Fi, WiMAX, ZigBee, Bluetooth, and LoRaWAN, among many others. A comprehensive survey and a performance comparative evaluation between them can be found in [59]. The integration of multiple devices exhibiting different IoT protocols makes data handling difficult, hinders their implementation, and slows down the communication capabilities thus reducing IoT scalability in healthcare.
3. **Network availability:** IoT relies on a communication network (Internet) to work. The availability of Internet might be evident in developed countries, but it might not be the case for developing economies. To successfully implement IoT-based healthcare solutions, both public and private sectors must commit to investing in an adequate infrastructure.

1.8 CONCLUSIONS

During the last years, the IoT paradigm has taken hold especially due to its characteristics associated with improving people's lives, easing decision making, and reducing the carbon footprint, among others.

This chapter has presented a holistic vision of the fundamentals of the IoT with the aim of providing a comprehensive overview to readers interested in the topic. The chapter has addressed the most relevant concepts involved in the IoT such as architectures, sensors, actuators, storage, communication protocols, and user interfaces. Finally, some IoT-based development applications for healthcare were provided. In this sense, it can be concluded that IoT can be successfully used in services related to patient monitoring, risky situations detection, telemedicine, among other applications.

REFERENCES

[1] K. Ashton, "That 'Internet of Things' Thing," *RFID J.*, p. 1, 2009.

[2] M. A. Medina C., "La historia detrás de la Internet de las Cosas," *El Espectador*, Bogotá, Oct. 05, 2017.

[3] C. Xiang and X. Li, "General Analysis on Architecture and Key Technologies about Internet of Things," in *ICSESS* 2012*: Proceedings of* 2012 *IEEE 3rd International Conference on Software Engineering and Service Science*, pp. 325–328, 2012.

[4] D. Evans, "The Internet of Things: How the Next Evolution of the Internet Is Changing Everything," *Cisco IBSG © 2011 Cisco and/or its affiliates*, 2011. http://www.cisco.com/web/about/ac79/docs/innov/IoT_IBSG_0411FINAL.pdf (accessed Jul. 19, 2020).

[5] International Telecommunication Union, "ITU work on Internet of Things," *ICTP Workshop*, 2015.

[6] J. Gubbi, R. Buyya, S. Marusic, and M. Palaniswami, "Internet of Things (IoT): A vision, architectural elements, and future directions," *Future Gener. Comput. Syst.*, vol. 29, no. 7, pp. 1645–1660, 2013, doi: 10.1016/j.future.2013.01.010.

[7] L. Atzori, A. Iera, and G. Morabito, "The Internet of Things: A survey," *Comput. Netw.*, vol. 54, no. 15, pp. 2787–2805, Oct. 2010, doi: 10.1016/j.comnet.2010.05.010.

[8] M. Jia, A. Komeily, Y. Wang, and R. S. Srinivasan, "Adopting Internet of Things for the development of smart buildings: A review of enabling technologies and applications," *Autom. Constr.*, vol. 101, pp. 111–126, Sep. 2019, doi: 10.1016/j.autcon.2019.01.023.

[9] R. Dobrescu, D. Merezeanu, and S. Mocanu, "Context-aware control and monitoring system with IoT and cloud support," *Comput. Electron. Agric.*, vol. 160, pp. 91–99, May 2019, doi: 10.1016/j.compag.2019.03.005.

[10] A. Khanna and S. Kaur, "Evolution of Internet of Things (IoT) and its significant impact in the field of Precision Agriculture," *Computers and Electronics in Agriculture*, vol. 157. Elsevier B.V., pp. 218–231, Feb. 01, 2019, doi: 10.1016/j.compag.2018.12.039.

[11] M. M. Komarov and M. D. Nemova, "Emerging of new service-oriented approach based on the Internet of Services and Internet of Things," in *Proceedings* - 2013 *IEEE 10th International Conference on e-Business Engineering, ICEBE* 2013, pp. 429–434, 2013, doi: 10.1109/ICEBE.2013.66.

[12] National Intelligence Council (NIC), "Disruptive Civil Technologies-Six Technologies With Potential Impacts on US Interests Out to 2025: CR2008-07," Washington (National Intelligence Council), 2008.

[13] M. Jia, A. Komeily, Y. Wang, and R. S. Srinivasan, "Adopting Internet of Things for the development of smart buildings: A review of enabling technologies and applications," *Autom. Constr.*, vol. 101, pp. 111–126, May 2019, doi: 10.1016/j.autcon.2019.01.023.

[14] R. Lanotte and M. Merro, "A semantic theory of the Internet of Things," *Inf. Comput.*, vol. 259, pp. 72–101, Apr. 2018, doi: 10.1016/j.ic.2018.01.001.

[15] A. Al-Fuqaha, M. Guizani, M. Mohammadi, M. Aledhari, and M. Ayyash, "Internet of Things: A survey on enabling technologies, protocols, and applications," *IEEE Commun. Surv. Tutor.*, vol. 17, no. 4, pp. 2347–2376, Oct. 2015, doi: 10.1109/COMST.2015.2444095.

[16] P. P. Ray, "A survey on Internet of Things architectures," *Journal of King Saud University - Computer and Information Sciences*, vol. 30, no. 3. King Saud bin Abdulaziz University, pp. 291–319, Jul. 01, 2018, doi: 10.1016/j.jksuci.2016.10.003.

[17] P. Pico-Valencia, J. A. Holgado-Terriza, and X. Quinonez-Ku, "A brief survey of the main internet-based approaches. An outlook from the internet of things perspective," in *Proceedings - 3rd International Conference on Information and Computer Technologies, ICICT* 2020, pp. 536–542, Mar. 2020, doi: 10.1109/ICICT50521.2020.00091.

[18] International Telecommunication Union, "Next Generation Networks-Frameworks and functional architecture models," 2012. http://handle.itu.int/11.1002/1000/1 (accessed Jul. 21, 2020).
[19] D. C. Yacchirema Vargas, "Arquitectura de interoperabilidad de dispositivos físicos para el internet de las cosas (IoT)," Universidad Politécnica de Valencia, 2019.
[20] A. Cobos Domínguez, "Diseño e implementación de una arquitectura IoT basada en tecnologías Open Source," Universidad de Sevilla, 2016.
[21] S. Kuyoro, F. Osisanwo, and O. Akinsowon, "Internet of Things (IoT): An Overview," in *3rd International Conference on Advances in Engineering Sciences & Applied Mathematics (ICAESAM'2015)*, pp. 53–58, Mar. 2015, doi: 10.15242/iie.e0315045.
[22] B. Dorsemaine, J. P. Gaulier, J. P. Wary, N. Kheir, and P. Urien, "Internet of Things: A Definition and Taxonomy," in *Proceedings - NGMAST* 2015*: The 9th International Conference on Next Generation Mobile Applications, Services and Technologies*, pp. 72–77, Jan. 2016, doi: 10.1109/NGMAST.2015.71.
[23] M. Wu, T. J. Lu, F. Y. Ling, J. Sun, and H. Y. Du, "Research on the architecture of Internet of Things," in *ICACTE* 2010 - 2010 *3rd International Conference on Advanced Computer Theory and Engineering, Proceedings*, vol. 5, 2010, doi: 10.1109/ICACTE.2010.5579493.
[24] C. W. Tsai, C. F. Lai and A. V. Vasilakos, "Future Internet of Things: open issues and challenges," *Wirel. Netw.*, vol. 20, no. 8, pp. 2201–2217, Oct. 2014, doi: 10.1007/s11276-014-0731-0.
[25] E. Borgia, "The Internet of Things vision: Key features, applications and open issues," *Computer Communications*, vol. 54. Elsevier, pp. 1–31, Dec. 01, 2014, doi: 10.1016/j.comcom.2014.09.008.
[26] S. Li, L. Da Xu and S. Zhao, "The Internet of Things: a survey," *Inf. Syst. Front.*, vol. 17, no. 2, pp. 243–259, 2015, doi: 10.1007/s10796-014-9492-7.
[27] D. Benítez, C. Anías, and L. Plasencia, "Propuesta de arquitectura para Internet de las Cosas," in *18 Convención Científica de Ingeniería y Arquitectura*, pp. 1–12, 2016.
[28] R. Khan, S. U. Khan, R. Zaheer, and S. Khan, "Future internet: The internet of things architecture, possible applications and key challenges," in *Proceedings - 10th International Conference on Frontiers of Information Technology, FIT* 2012, pp. 257–260, 2012, doi: 10.1109/FIT.2012.53.
[29] C. M. de Morais, D. Sadok, and J. Kelner, "An IoT sensor and scenario survey for data researchers," *J. Braz. Comput. Soc.*, vol. 25, no. 1, p. 4, Feb. 2019, doi: 10.1186/s13173-019-0085-7.
[30] P. P. Ray, "A survey on Internet of Things architectures," *J. King Saud Univ. - Comput. Inf. Sci.*, vol. 30, no. 3, pp. 291–319, Jul. 2018, doi: 10.1016/j.jksuci.2016.10.003.
[31] M. F. Kamaruzaman, N. M. Rani, H. M. Nor, and M. H. H. Azahari, "Developing user interface design application for children with autism," *Procedia - Soc. Behav. Sci.*, vol. 217, pp. 887–894, Feb. 2016, doi: 10.1016/j.sbspro.2016.02.022.
[32] A. Darejeh and D. Singh, "A review on user interface design principles to increase software usability for users with less computer literacy," *J. Comput. Sci.*, vol. 9, no. 11, pp. 1443–1450, Nov. 2013, doi: 10.3844/jcssp.2013.1443.1450.
[33] T. Alves, J. Natálio, J. Henriques-Calado, and S. Gama, "Incorporating personality in user interface design: A review," *Personal. Individ. Differ.*, vol. 155, p. 109709, Mar. 2020, doi: 10.1016/j.paid.2019.109709.
[34] L. Ratcliffe and S. Puthusserypady, "Importance of Graphical User Interface in the design of P300 based Brain–Computer Interface systems," *Comput. Biol. Med.*, vol. 117, p. 103599, Feb. 2020, doi: 10.1016/j.compbiomed.2019.103599.
[35] L.-H. Chen and Y.-C. Liu, "Affordance and intuitive interface design for elder users with dementia," *Procedia CIRP*, vol. 60, pp. 470–475, Jan. 2017, doi: 10.1016/j.procir.2017.02.015.

[36] A. R. Al-Ali, I. A. Zualkernan, M. Rashid, R. Gupta, and M. Alikarar, "A smart home energy management system using IoT and big data analytics approach," *IEEE Trans. Consum. Electron.*, vol. 63, no. 4, pp. 426–434, Nov. 2017, doi: 10.1109/TCE.2017.015014.

[37] M. Villalpando, R. V. Guerrero and P. A. G. Mier, "Sistemas de telediagnóstico: Maletín médico de ingeniería aplicada," *Rev. Mex. Ing. Bioméd.*, vol. 22, no. 2, pp. 107–113, 2001.

[38] R. Velazquez, "An optimal adaptive filtering approach for stress-tests motion artifacts removal: application on an ECG for telediagnosis," in *6th International Conference on Signal Processing,* vol. 2, pp. 1504–1507, 2002.

[39] R. Fensli, E. Gunnarson, and T. Gundersen, "A wearable ECG-recording system for continuous arrhythmia monitoring in a wireless tele-home-care situation," in *18th IEEE Symposium on Computer-Based Medical Systems (CBMS'05)*, pp. 407–412, 2005.

[40] B. Kutlu, A. Kut, and M. Yildirim, "Tele-health monitoring platform," in 2010 *15th National Biomedical Engineering Meeting*, pp. 1–4, Apr. 2010, doi: 10.1109/BIYOMUT.2010.5479732.

[41] Z. Zhang, T.-P. Jung, S. Makeig, and B. D. Rao, "Compressed sensing of EEG for wireless telemonitoring with low energy consumption and inexpensive hardware," *IEEE Trans. Biomed. Eng.*, vol. 60, no. 1, pp. 221–224, Jan. 2013, doi: 10.1109/TBME.2012.2217959.

[42] R. Mahajan and D. Bansal, "Hybrid multichannel EEG compression scheme for tele-health monitoring," in *Infocom Technologies and Optimization Proceedings of 3rd International Conference on Reliability*, pp. 1–6, Oct. 2014, doi: 10.1109/ICRITO.2014.7014672.

[43] R. Ciobotariu, C. Rotariu, F. Adochiei, and H. Costin, "Wireless breathing system for long term telemonitoring of respiratory activity," in *7th International Symposium on Advanced Topics in Electrical Engineering*, pp. 1–4, May 2011.

[44] M. Vishwaracharya and R. Mohan, "Implementation of a wearable cardiorespiratory monitoring device," in *IEEE Region 10 Conference (TENCON)*, pp. 344–349, Nov. 2016, doi: 10.1109/TENCON.2016.7848018.

[45] A. Hariton, L. Nita, and M. Cretu, "A web application for blood glucose monitoring using the iPhone advantages," in *International Conference and Exposition on Electrical and Power Engineering*, pp. 505–508, Oct. 2012, doi: 10.1109/ICEPE.2012.6463883.

[46] R. S. H. Istepanian, A. Sungoor, and K. A. Earle, "Technical and compliance considerations for mobile health self-monitoring of glucose and blood pressure for patients with diabetes," in *Annual International Conference of the IEEE Engineering in Medicine and Biology Society*, pp. 5130–5133, Sep. 2009, doi: 10.1109/IEMBS.2009.5334580.

[47] H. Jian and H. Chen, "A portable fall detection and alerting system based on k-NN algorithm and remote medicine," *China Commun.*, vol. 12, no. 4, pp. 23–31, Apr. 2015, doi: 10.1109/CC.2015.7114066.

[48] N. Kattukkaran, A. George, and T. P. M. Haridas, "Intelligent accident detection and alert system for emergency medical assistance," in *International Conference on Computer Communication and Informatics (ICCCI)*, pp. 1–6, Jan. 2017, doi: 10.1109/ICCCI.2017.8117791.

[49] A. Pawlak, K. Horoba, J. Jezewski, J. Wrobel, and A. Matonia, "Telemonitoring of pregnant women at home — Biosignals acquisition and measurement," in *22nd International Conference Mixed Design of Integrated Circuits Systems (MIXDES)*, pp. 83–87, Jun. 2015, doi: 10.1109/MIXDES.2015.7208486.

[50] P. Kuwik, T. Largi, M. York, D. Crump, D. Livingston, and J. C. Squire, "The smart medical refrigerator," *IEEE Potentials*, vol. 24, no. 1, pp. 42–45, Feb. 2005, doi: 10.1109/MP.2005.1405802.

[51] R. Velázquez, E. Pissaloux, P. Rodrigo, M. Carrasco, N. I. Giannoccaro, and A. Lay-Ekuakille, "An Outdoor Navigation System for Blind Pedestrians Using GPS and Tactile-Foot Feedback," *Appl. Sci.*, vol. 8, no. 4, Art. no. 4, Apr. 2018, doi: 10.3390/app8040578.

[52] E. Pissaloux and R. Velázquez, "Model of Cognitive Mobility for Visually Impaired and its Experimental Validation," in *Mobility of Visually Impaired People: Fundamentals and ICT Assistive Technologies*, E. Pissaloux and R. Velazquez, Eds. Cham: Springer International Publishing, pp. 311–352, 2018.

[53] "OpenStreetMap Project," 2020. https://www.openstreetmap.org/ (accessed Jul. 24, 2020).

[54] "YOURS map and router-finder," June 2020. http://yournavigation.org/ (accessed Jul. 24, 2020).

[55] R. Velázquez and E. Pissaloux, "On human performance in tactile language learning and tactile memory," in *The 23rd IEEE International Symposium on Robot and Human Interactive Communication*, pp. 96–101, Aug. 2014, doi: 10.1109/ROMAN.2014.6926236.

[56] C.-Y. Su, C.-Y. Hsiao, R.-G. Lee, and J.-H. Chen, "TaoBall: An interactive IoT ball design for rehabilitation," in 2016 *IEEE 6th International Conference on Consumer Electronics - Berlin (ICCE-Berlin)*, pp. 24–27, Sep. 2016, doi: 10.1109/ICCE-Berlin.2016.7684708.

[57] K. C. Yang, C. H. Huang, and C.-Y. ChiangLin, "Combining IOT and Android APP System for Upper Limb Stroke Rehabilitation," in *IEEE International Conference on Industrial Engineering and Engineering Management (IEEM)*, pp. 1096–1100, Dec. 2018, doi: 10.1109/IEEM.2018.8607742.

[58] A. Sula, E. Spaho, K. Matsuo, L. Barolli, R. Miho, and F. Xhafa, "An IoT-Based System for Supporting Children with Autism Spectrum Disorder," in 2013 *Eighth International Conference on Broadband and Wireless Computing, Communication and Applications*, pp. 282–289, Oct. 2013, doi: 10.1109/BWCCA.2013.51.

[59] C. Del-Valle-Soto, L. J. Valdivia, R. Velázquez, L. Rizo-Dominguez, and J.-C. López-Pimentel, "Smart campus: An experimental performance comparison of collaborative and cooperative schemes for Wireless Sensor Network," *Energies*, vol. 12, no. 16, Art. no. 16, Jan. 2019, doi: 10.3390/en12163135.

2 Internet of Medical Things: *Current and Future Trends*

Lucia Alonso Virgos[1], Miguel A. Sanchez Vidales[2], Fernando López Hernández[3], and J. Javier Rainer Granados[4]
[1-4]Universidad International de la Rioja (UNIR), Av. de la Paz 136, 26006, Logroño, Spain

CONTENTS

2.1 Introduction 20
2.2 Use of Robotics in Medicine 21
 2.2.1 Robotic Surgery 21
 2.2.2 Robots for Rehabilitation and Prosthesis 21
 2.2.3 Robots for Storage and Distribution of Drugs 22
 2.2.4 Benefits of Robots in Healthcare 22
 2.2.5 Disadvantages of Robots in Healthcare 22
 2.2.6 Future Trends in Robotics 23
2.3 Data-Driven Medicine 23
 2.3.1 Purpose of the Studies 23
 2.3.2 Types of Studies 24
 2.3.3 Exposure Measurement 24
 2.3.4 Ethical Issues 25
 2.3.5 Future Trends in Data-Driven Medicine 25
2.4 Image Management and Video Surveillance Applied in Medicine 25
 2.4.1 Imaging Modalities 25
 2.4.2 Classical Postprocessing Techniques 26
 2.4.3 Segmentation 27
 2.4.4 3D Reconstruction and Registration 27
 2.4.5 Medical Video Surveillance 27
 2.4.6 Future Trends in Image Processing 28
2.5 Cybersecurity: The Need for Security in Medical it Systems 28
 2.5.1 Future Trends in Cybersecurity 29

2.6 Legislation Applied to Iomt in Medicine....29
2.6.1 Legislation in Europe....29
2.6.2 Three Scenarios in Data Protection....30
2.6.3 Future Trends in Legislation....31
2.7 Conclusions....32
References....33

2.1 INTRODUCTION

Nowadays, all kinds of small devices, called "things", have computing features. For this reason, the label "smart" is added to phones, clothes, cars, and home appliances. In addition, the Internet and the broadband and wireless networks make possible performing complex and very useful solutions in every field. In medicine, these advances and technologies are very important. The Internet of Medical Things (IoMT) establishes the necessary scenario to interconnect and manage these smart medical devices or things, like scanners, analyzers, wearables, sensors or operating material.

Because of that, now we can store, manage and compute huge amounts of data and images to perform better diagnostics, and using Artificial Intelligence (AI) techniques, we can also predict epidemics. Using video surveillance, it is possible to improve the interaction with remote patients. In addition, with advanced robots, a surgeon can perform an operation in a much more precise and secure way. And, in some cases, these technologies are combined and related to design better solutions; e.g., a team of surgeons in different countries can use video surveillance to guide and perform an operation and remotely control the robot used in an operation, making medical decisions based on advanced image processing and Big Data.

Taking all of this into account, in this chapter we will analyze some of the most relevant current and future trends referred to as the IoMT. Specifically, we will address the following:

1. Robotics. Robotics are becoming more and more important because they can improve on and provide some key benefits such as high precision, lower risks, better prosthesis or better and faster recovery times after robotic surgery.
2. Data-driven medicine. Today, there are huge databases with medical information on millions of people. Due to this fact, it is possible to make automatic analysis that facilitates the forecasting of epidemics.
3. Image analysis and video surveillance. Medical imaging assists a doctor in detecting the state and extent of a disease without any surgery. These technologies, in many cases, are closely related to other topics like robotics, e.g., to register images in an automated scanner, wearables; to retrieve and visualize diagrams of personal measurement data or data-driven medicine; and to generate graphics with trends. The patients can be remotely monitored using video surveillance equipment [1, 2].

4. Cybersecurity. In all the previous points, security is one of the aspects that most concern the field of IoMT.
5. Legislation. The main objective of the regulation is to create a culture of data protection in health issues. For this reason, we discuss the main points of data protection covered by the European legislation.

The objective is to offer a theoretical framework that allows one to initiate new lines of research focused on offering new methods and/or analyzing carefully the benefits, the methods of implementation and the evaluation of each one of the existing systems.

2.2 USE OF ROBOTICS IN MEDICINE

Robotics is of great utility in medicine. Its automation and high precision give specialists access to areas of risk or areas where any error might be fatal. Besides offering an improved intervention, this technology helps with faster recovery for patients. Robotics does not damage the healthy tissues that are near the operation area; also avoids involuntary movements during surgery. In addition to being present during an operation, a robot can also assist a patient with alternatives to a prosthesis or distribution of drugs; which is required mostly in patients who do not react and are in critical situations. Therefore, healthcare robotics is classified into three assistance stages: (a) Robotic surgery, (b) robots for rehabilitation and prosthesis, and (c) robots for storage and distribution of drugs.

2.2.1 Robotic Surgery

This type of robots assists surgeons in performing complex interventions with very positive results (e.g., [3]). These interventions might be related to accuracy or strength; for example, surgery in the head or the cerebral area where precision and accuracy play a crucial role. On the other hand, an example of strength-related intervention is the case of cutting a bone in such a way that healthy areas do not get damaged, such as tissues or the rest of the bone. Robotic surgery helps to obtain higher accuracy in the process, decrease time of operation, decrease time of wound healing and therefore recovery time. The robot can be guided by cameras and with the appropriate information about the patient, it can fulfill different functions; for example, this technology might change according to the need, ranging from a conventional mechanical arm up to elements of measurement. Also, advantages of remote surgery should be underscored, as it allows patients to receive a better treatment when any specialist from across the globe can assist in surgery or in offering advice.

2.2.2 Robots for Rehabilitation and Prosthesis

With this type of robots, the patient obtains therapy more adapted to rehabilitation (e.g., [4]) because this technology helps the therapist perform the right movements and with the appropriate strength according to the medical prognosis. Also it is a very useful tool for therapists, as a major concern nowadays is studying in depth the methods for a better patient recovery rather than the correct movement of the affected area. On the robotic prosthesis side, science keeps advancing. There are available prostheses that can respond to the patient's wills sent by the patient's brain to perform a movement through the prosthesis. These signals that the patient sends from the brain are called myoelectric signals.

2.2.3 Robots for Storage and Distribution of Drugs

Doctors in hospitals and clinics are responsible for preparing a precise list of drugs to supply to their patients (e.g., [5]). However, it is hard to keep track of schedules and exact doses taking into account the number of patients that are in a care center at one time. This explains the utility of robotics because due to its accuracy, it provides higher control of the doses and the exact hours in which every patient receives drugs, which will obviously help in the recovery of the patient. This is also necessary for patients with more severe illnesses, those who need accurate control, and for patients who are weak or immobile.

2.2.4 Benefits of Robots in Healthcare

We have seen now that nowadays robotics is a very important tool; therefore, I will list some advantages that we can obtain from this technology in the healthcare industry:

a. Robots deliver major safety, accuracy, and precision when performing an intervention in a patient.
b. With the robotics technology, operations are shorter and recovery time is cut greatly because the wounds diminish due to the efficacy of the robots in operations.
c. It is possible to perform interventions by teleoperation (telesurgery), reducing travel costs, increasing efficiency and improving the quality of surgical procedures.
d. Surgeons using robotics can perform cuts without damaging the healthy parts.
e. Unlike human beings, robots do not show fear, weariness or fatigue; therefore, they can operate indefinitely and always using the best way.
f. Remote surgery results in an assisted or advised intervention by any specialist around the globe.
g. Nowadays, the loss of any extremity is not a handicap since very high-quality robotic prostheses can be supplied.
h. Using robots for storage and distribution of drugs, we can have much more suitable and exact monitoring at the time of giving the medication.

2.2.5 Disadvantages of Robots in Healthcare

Currently, there are very few disadvantages of using robots in healthcare, as follows:

a. The intervention is much more expensive with robots than the conventional way.

b. At present, it is not possible to operate on children who weigh under 20 pounds; although this will change soon with the upcoming advances in technology.
c. More time is needed in the programming stage to obtain the wished results.

2.2.6 Future Trends in Robotics

We all know that technology is in continuous progress. The capability of nanobots to perform surveillance is one of the most attractive future trends in robotics [5]. Since ancient times, scientists have been dreaming of small machines that could realize unimaginable works. The physicist Richard Feynman was the first one who thought about the possibility of having these benefits from very small machines. The main characteristic of the nanorobots or nanobots is that their size is less than one nanometer.

Nowadays, the National Aeronautics and Space Administration (NASA) is the most advanced organization in the study of nanotechnology, the importance lies in the use that nanotechnology has to improve the resistance of spacecraft.

The need that man has to survive in zero gravity or the pressures of outer space makes NASA scientists research and develop applications of nanotechnology in health. In addition, being small devices, they can enter a person's body without hurting them to fight against bacteria, viruses, toxins and even specific cells.

2.3 DATA-DRIVEN MEDICINE

Nowadays medical services have huge databases with the longitudinal medical records of millions of people. The question that researchers are addressing is to what extent the automatic analysis of these databases facilitates the forecasting of epidemics [6]. This data-driven medicine will help the health authorities achieve better prevention, provision of resources and significant savings in hospitalization costs. Furthermore, this means an increase in the life expectancy of the population. In this section we will review the current status of these techniques.

2.3.1 Purpose of the Studies

Clinical epidemiology aims to demonstrate epidemiological causality based on medical studies. Epidemiology is used here in a broad sense, that is, it does not only address infectious diseases, but risk factors such as smoking, BMI, etc.

The purpose of epidemiological studies can be divided into surveillance and prediction [7]. Surveillance monitors the state of the disease in the time, the place or the risk group, in order to orient the development of public health programs. Prediction aims to discover new associations (epidemiological hypothesis) between exposures and diseases.

2.3.2 Types of Studies

The underlying studies have been traditionally classified into observational and experimental studies [8]. Observational studies do not expose participants to the risk factors; the most common observational types are:

1. **Case study** surveys the evolution of a particular individual suffering from a certain disease, within a particular situation or period of time.
2. **Case-control study** is a retrospective survey of two groups: one with the disease (the case) and another one without the disease (the control). Typically, the odds ratio between the exposure levels of both groups is measured aiming to determine the level of causality between the exposure and the disease.
3. **Cohort study** is a longitudinal study that samples a cohort (group of individuals at risk of developing the disease) [9]. The study registers through time the level of exposure of the individuals to the risk factors and those who have developed the disease.

In experimental studies, the researcher manipulates the level of exposure of the participants to a drug or to a risk factor. The most common study is the clinical trial in which some participants are given a drug, and others a placebo. The objective is to conclude whether the effect of the drug is statistically significant.

2.3.3 Exposure Measurement

Exposure measurement gauges the level of exposition of the participants by means of regular medical tests and questionnaires. The IoMT has given rise to a set of wearable devices that facilitate the precise monitoring of the vital signs. For instance, [10] describes its use to monitor stress levels throughout the day. These measures allow determining the level of association between the exposure (explanatory factor) and the response. The more obvious inherent difficulties are the bias (i.e., systematic error) and precision (i.e., random error) of the measurements. However, there are other major difficulties that frequently cause misleading conclusions:

1. **Confounders** are disregarded variables that modify the weight of the association between the exposure and the observed response, or cause spurious associations. For example, when studying how the consumption of alcohol (exposure) affects the BMI (response), the researcher can be ignoring confounding variables such as whether the alcohol consumers are paying less attention to their diet. The authors of [11] describe a number of techniques to decrease the occurrence of confounding.
2. **Heterogeneity** occurs when different groups may have different levels of response to the exposure factor. For example, men have a significatively lower incidence of breast cancer than women. If we do not separate the participant by sex, what we will obtain is a weighted average of the response. One approach to deal with heterogeneous responses is stratification, which

partitions the cases whenever we think that gender is altering the results. Stratification facilitates comparison, but it is important to ensure that all the subgroups are sufficiently represented in the sample.

3. **Interactions** frequently occur applying techniques such as analysis of variance or regression analysis. In particular, they occur if there is an exposure to several risk factors, and the contribution of the risk factors is not additive, but multiplicative. For instance, gender interacts with other risk factors accentuating or decreasing the occurrence of breast cancer.

2.3.4 Ethical Issues

Ethical issues arise when instead of using datasets to prevent diseases, they can also be used for other purposes; for instance, to choose or discard the clients of an insurer, or to decide on the granting of mortgages. Therefore, to prevent abuses, we have to be vigilant about the purpose for which the above-mentioned techniques are being used.

2.3.5 Future Trends in Data-Driven Medicine

A challenge that is still unresolved is in data munging. Clinical records are very messy and include missing values, outliers, etc. Consequently, there must exist a preprocessing step that mixes and reorders the data before their injection into a classification or prediction algorithm. Unfortunately, this process is still done manually and is extremely tedious. A line of contribution to this area is the use of imputation techniques for handling missing data[6]].

A second area of improvement is the use of machine understating to improve the prediction accuracy. We think that nowadays it is difficult to advance the (already highly developed) statistical techniques, without the ability of the machine to understand the implications of the data, in a similar way that humans develop intuitions from manual data inspection.

2.4 IMAGE MANAGEMENT AND VIDEO SURVEILLANCE APPLIED IN MEDICINE

When a doctor needs to know the status of a patient, a picture is worth a thousand words. Medical imaging assists the doctor to detect the state and extent of a disease without any surgery. In fact, the capture and processing of images of the human body is nowadays ubiquitous in medicine.

2.4.1 Imaging Modalities

Before analyzing a medical image, it is necessary to capture it. The most common techniques for capturing medical images of the body's interior are described below:

1. **Sonography** consists in emitting ultrasounds that are propagated by the body to be analyzed. Ultrasounds are well transmitted by water, but produce

echoes when finding bones, calcifications or fat. Although the images are not as clear as in other approaches, this technique has the advantage of not having risks.

2. **Magnetic Resonance Images (MRI)** measures radio frequency signals emitted by hydrogen when it resonates with strong magnetic fields. This technique is very popular because it allows you to capture clear images without the need to expose the body to radiation.
3. **Functional Magnetic Resonance Imaging (fMRI)** is a popular MRI application to measure the brain activity. Specifically, the technique detects increases in blood flow in areas of the brain that are activated. In this way, it is possible to know which parts of the brain are involved in each cognitive activity.
4. **Positron Emission Tomography (PET)** uses small amounts of radioactive material that the patient must swallow, and which acts as a tracer. The use of substances with certain biochemical reactions (for example glucose) allows concentrating the radioactive material in certain parts of the body. This technique is very precise and so it can be used to capture both macroscopic and microscopic images.
5. **Computed Tomography (CT).** It is possible to create a set of virtually scanned sliced images (typically PET or MRI) to obtain a 3D reconstruction of an organ.
6. **X-ray Imaging** is one of the oldest and most frequent techniques due to its ease of use and the clarity of the captured images. It consists in circulating gamma radiations through the body. Solid structures such as bones have a higher absorption rate than liquids. This contrast appears in the image collected on a plate on the other side of the emitter.

2.4.2 Classical Postprocessing Techniques

Once the images have been captured, different image postprocessing techniques are used to enhance them. The most basic, classic and effective techniques are:

1. **Histogram equalization.** This technique increases the overall contrast of an image by redistributing the intensity levels of the histogram [12].
2. **Deblurring.** We can use standard techniques of contrast enhancement to increase the clarity of the blurred areas of a medical image (see, for example, [13]).
3. **Thresholding.** This technique converts a gray-level image into a binary image. Therefore, it acts as an easy binary classification technique. For instance, [14] describes a method to select the optimum threshold value for medical images.
4. **Combination of images.** By combining different images, you can retrieve information lost in the individual images. For example, [15] proposes a method to combine PER and MRI images.

5. **Edges and boundaries detection.** These techniques aim at identifying parts of an image in which color or brightness changes sharply. For instance, [16] describes a method to accurately detect prostate boundaries in an ultrasound image.

Below we describe other more advanced techniques, which frequently rely on these basic ones.

2.4.3 Segmentation

This technique aims to automatically label the regions of the image to ease the selection of the object of interest in the image (e.g., [5, 6]). See [17] for a review of segmentation techniques in medicine. Segmentation can be divided into:

1. **Region-based segmentation**, which assumes that neighboring pixels have similar properties, in terms of intensity, color, texture, etc. For instance, [18] describes a method to segment the regions corresponding to melanoma skin cancer.
2. **Boundary-based segmentation**, which assumes that the properties of the pixels change abruptly at the boundaries of the object. This corresponds to the idea of membrane in biology.

2.4.4 3D Reconstruction and Registration

Modern CT techniques are able to reconstruct a 3D image from multiple sliced images. For instance, in diagnosis, the area affected by a tumor can be reconstructed in 3D to guide surgical removal.

Registration is the process of mapping a 3D object to a set of 2D captured images. For instance, [19] describes a method to delineate the 3D left ventricle from a set of MRI images. Usually, the registration involves identifying the translations, rotations and scaling necessary to match the 3D identified object. A well-known difficulty in medicine is that the organs are not rigid, but deformable. Therefore, a set of posed consistency methods has been developed [20].

2.4.5 Medical Video Surveillance

Medical video surveillance is becoming a necessary service in the safety plans of health centers, but the decision to use video surveillance can bring controversy. On the one hand, it can be useful to protect the patient and to protect the equipment. On the other hand, the privacy of the patient may be under attack. Taking that into account during a medical consultation, privacy must be a priority and video surveillance must be carefully treated.

According to European law, health centers can capture images through video cameras to preserve the safety of people and property. These images must be removed within a maximum period of one month, unless they must be made available to a competent authority within a maximum period of 72 hours [7]. If the images were to be sent to the competent authority, IoMT is also needed, specifically used motion sensors, telephone consoles, panic buttons, magnetic contacts, alarm, etc. [13].

The tendency is to find a balance between compliance with legislation and the protection of patient privacy by suggesting mechanisms that reassure authorities, professionals, and patients at the same time.

2.4.6 Future Trends in Image Processing

There are several unsolved challenges in medical imaging. The first challenge is that 3D reconstruction is an ill-posed problem. This means that we can get several 3D reconstructions from a set of 2D images. To manage this difficulty, the so-called regularization techniques aim to limit or minimize the error.

A second challenge is the use of a medical image, not just to diagnose, but also to accomplish automatic/semiautomatic robotic surgery. For example, by using miniaturized robots that move through the veins.

A third challenge is virtual reality surgery simulation, which facilitates training surgeons before conducting real interventions.

2.5 CYBERSECURITY: THE NEED FOR SECURITY IN MEDICAL IT SYSTEMS

It is relatively common for healthcare centers to use a network infrastructure. These devices are connected both in the rooms of the hospital and the homes of patients. From the healthcare center itself, many profiles can be connected to the same network, so it is not easy to do Network Access Control (NAC), and there may be a vulnerability in the service.

However, there are new generation protocols that help protect data in IoT systems; for example, ZigBee. ZigBee is a set of wireless communication protocols aiming to connect applications with a low data rate. It is especially used in Wireless Sensor Networks (WSNs) for healthcare using medical radio bands (or ISM band) [21]; for example, to safely and reliably monitor diseases, home nursing, glucose meters, oxygen, blood pressure, etc.. It also helps create information management and visualization indicators [22]. ZigBee is a simple, economical and energy efficient technology [23]. The security systems offered are secure in communication, key management, and cryptography through three types of keys according to the network (master key, link key, and network key). Its weaknesses are its limited resources in the nodes, the low calculation capacity and the low memory they offer [21].

Despite the existence of protocols, security is one of the aspects that most concern the field of IoMT. This is because the less human interaction exists in the integration of the physical and digital world, the greater the efficiency, but also the greater the vulnerability to non-compliance with protection regulations (e.g., during cryptography). Authentication can pose an additional difficulty in the field of telemedicine. Another problem that the IoMT can bring with it during the use of medical devices is the saturation of data stored in a cloud. When this occurs, data exchange is almost impossible without applying infrequent prevention techniques in health contexts [24].

There are also the possibility of theft, manipulation during monitoring, espionage or attacks to the service, and situations in which the data may be compromised by cybercriminals. The violation of these medical devices causes free access to medical and/or personal information that can control the dispensing of medicine or even attacks to assistance robots [25].

Although in health services it is more common for insecurity to be caused by carelessness, ignorance of legislation or lack of digital maturity, the truth is that the patient in a medical service center is connected to devices through a wireless network, which makes it vulnerable. [25, 26].

2.5.1 Future Trends in Cybersecurity

In general, a service that bases its main action on the analysis and treatment of data can bring failures or breaches if they are not organized properly. These failures or breaches can trigger citizen protection problems. So, it is not surprising that as society advances, so should advancing the regulation on protection. The problem could be divided into two parts: the vulnerability of the devices discussed previously, and knowledge about the relevant legislation. For the first part, the future trends in cybersecurity will, for sure, increase the protection of these devices. For the second part, in the next section we introduce the main concepts about current and future trends about legislation.

2.6 LEGISLATION APPLIED TO IoMT IN MEDICINE

Workers in the healthcare sector may want to comply with the legislation, but they may not know of it or the adequate devices for its correct compliance. This can cause legal problems and trigger workers to fear possible consequences and be more cautious in their medical capabilities due to limited digital control.

The main objective of the regulation is to create a culture of data protection in health matters. The main goal is to prevent non-compliance and strengthen patient protection.

2.6.1 Legislation in Europe

In May 2016, Regulation (EU) 2016/679, General Data Protection Regulation (GDPR) was approved, which aims to unify the regimes of all the member states of the European Parliament. As of 2018, a series of mechanisms to protect the privacy and security of the citizen is mandatory. A few months later, the Organic Law 3/2018 of December 5, on Data Protection and Guarantee of Digital Rights was published in Spain. Among its most outstanding articles, those that can be directly linked to the IoMT in the healthcare field are:

a. **General obligations of the person responsible for data processing.** It is necessary that the healthcare centers have a figure that safeguards the treatment of the data. Patients must be protected from situations that may generate discrimination, identity theft or fraud, financial losses, damage to their reputation, loss of confidentiality, etc. art. 1 [27]. Impact assessments on privacy should be organized to determine the risks posed by the treatment according to which data, art. 91 [28]. In addition to protecting personal data, data on past, present or future health should be protected; art. 35 [28] regulates the assistance, tests or exams, medical history, and treatments.

b. **Profiling.** Profiling based on the personal data of a patient involves evaluating aspects related to their health, including personal fitness trackers, electronic measurements, other medical records, etc. IBM developed Watson, a useful intelligent system in the healthcare sector. One of its main objectives is the diagnostic service, improving accuracy up to 40%. This is known as cognitive computing. However, not all data that could be useful can be used by health devices. So, part of this information, mainly the information collected by the patient, ends up discarded. On the other hand, the information that is collected in healthcare centers is not always accessible to the patient [9]. According to European and Spanish regulations, children deserve specific protection of their data during the creation of profiles. This protection focuses on the use of data for marketing, personality characteristics, etc., art. 38 [28]. Automated decisions and profiling based on particular categories of personal data should only be allowed under specific conditions. Appropriate mathematical or statistical procedures should be used for profiling, applying appropriate technical and organizational measures to ensure that inaccuracies in personal data are corrected and the risk of error is minimized, art. 71 [28]. The trend in profiling should be a context where healthcare professionals and patients can legally share information relevant to their needs [29].

c. **Processing, transfer, and storage of data.** More and more chronically ill patients request home care. In these cases, cloud computing services can be used. This new form of data treatment provides the patients improved communication with the healthcare professionals who attend to them, sharing information regarding data, measurements and current records. However, this data collection may suffer from credibility. It is for this reason that there is danger in the transfer of patient data to the healthcare professional.

2.6.2 Three Scenarios in Data Protection

Healthcare centers also keep updated records of tests performed in their centers. This can cause three scenarios:

1. **No consent or understanding on the part of the patient.**
   This situation implies that the patient does not consent or is unaware of the storage of this information, especially when this information may be public in some wayIn this case, it is necessary to know that the visibility of the data must be authorized except where public interest is involved for purposes of security, supervision and public health alert, arts. 45 and 52 [28]. For example, this happens with serious communicable diseases.

In the same way, the processing of personal data without the consent of the interested party may be necessary for reasons of public interest. This treatment must be subject to appropriate and specific measures in order to protect the rights and freedoms of natural persons. In that context, 'public health' must be interpreted in the definition of Regulation (EC) No. 1338/2008 of the European Parliament and of the Council, art. 54 [28, 30].

If it is not in these public safety contexts, the patients can manifest their will through technological means, such as networks, applications, etc. Technology facilitates this type of communication. The consent at a distance must be able to guarantee the authenticity of the interested party and filter the minimum requirements that are required, arts. 6 and 7 [27]. For example, we must ensure that if the patient is under 14 years of age there is a titular figure which protects his rights as a minor.

Finally, the principles of fair and transparent treatment require the patient to be informed about the treatment of their data, art. 60 [28].

2. **Patient access to your data.**

As indicated in the previous section, the medical tests carried out in healthcare centers generate data stored in these centers. Although the patient must trust that these data cannot put at risk the rights and freedoms of patients, according to art. [28], in many cases patients demand access to their records, but there is not any available access mechanism.

With the new legislation, interested patients must have the right to access their data. If possible, the controller should be able to provide remote access to a secure system that offers the patients concerned direct access to their personal data, art. 63 [28].

3. **Data transfer.**

Sharing data not only helps the healthcare professional but can be useful for the healthcare community. This occurs when the information may be relevant for specific issues, such as a change in the patient's residence. The automatic transfer of data allows the patients not to have to request such data and healthcare services can interchange the medical history of patients with other centers. The patient's interest is protected if there is disagreement, as indicated in art. 112 [28].

On the other hand, sharing data can boost scientific research. If the result of the investigation can benefit the patient, the objective of the TFEU reserved for this matter must be taken into account, art. 159 [28, 31].

2.6.3 Future Trends in Legislation

Fulfilling these requirements and creating an environment of transparency generate a state of trust between patients and healthcare centers. The current trend in the treatment, transfer, and storage of data could be the creation of a tool that helps healthcare centers to effectively use medical devices linked to the IoMT. There are guides for evaluation of the impact on the protection of personal data. The advantage is that professionals can identify possible risks in the protection of patient data so that they can be corrected [32].

The future trend that can improve these guides is possibly training. It is useful to combine technology, legislation, and health in the same field, but also training.

In a context where training is integrated into all IoMT fields, there would be no security deficiencies, because technology would provide legal knowledge to medical devices and documentation about their use and the need to meet safety requirements for healthcare professionals.

Proper communication and anti-stall automation can also be useful. Although all three fields are trained and familiar with the knowledge that concerns others, there is a risk of making mistakes. With fluid communication betweenservices and legislation, and between legislation and technology, these failures can be anticipated and minimized.

2.7 CONCLUSIONS

In this chapter we have analyzed some of the most important subjects of the Internet of Medical Things (IoMT): robotics, data-driven medicine, image analysis and video surveillance, cybersecurity, and legislation. In these IoMT fields, we have described current and future trends that could be the basis of a theoretical framework for new research lines.

We have described how robotics has several benefits and alternatives; it has permitted human beings to have many different solutions to daily problems. Robotics has encouraged a lot of expectations in the medical field; as we have seen, there are many advantages such as speed, accuracy, precision and above everything, more efficient work to improve our health and our iterations in it. With this technology, it has become possible to reach places of our anatomy that were very difficult to access in a way that gives specialists a higher success level in their work. Robotics also offers patients more confidence in accepting any type of intervention, be it complex or very risky.

In the field of data-driven medicine, the automatic processing of massive clinical data allows performing large-scale simulations, predicting how diseases could evolve, and understanding what interventions would be most effective.

In other areas, medical imaging techniques enable the visualization of the interior of the human body so that the surgeon can make decisions in a non-invasive way. These images are also useful to educate doctors in training and open the doors to automatic/semiautomatic robotic surgery.

Finally, cybersecurity and legislation probably are and will be one of the most important subjects with regard to IoMT. Security and data protection in IoT in healthcare involves legislation, technology, and health; it would be interesting for the three fields to be unified.

The legislation is fundamental to create a preventive culture on data protection, but applied to technology it can bring harm to the system. Healthcare must be up-to-date on matters related to digital protection, and its devices must include resources that promote digital maturity.

In addition, safety is an aspect of life that allows people to have confidence. In medicine, it is important that patients feel far from any danger or threat. Even if patients trust the professionals for their medical competencies, they also need to be sure of their privacy.

There are many circumstances why this privacy may be violated. Technological advances can pose an even greater danger to this possible violation of privacy. In particular because the devices are capable of storing, sharing and generating so much data that a human being is not able to control.

Healthcare workers are unaware that there is such a violation because they are experts in medicine, not legislation. It is important that technology communicates with the legislation during the development of devices. And that the legislation is within reach of the knowledge of services, in case there are security failures in said devices.

IoMT is still learning from its experience, but it is going in the right direction and will be able to contribute to the existence of a social context in which there is no lack of security.

It is mutually beneficial to have health and technology working together, because the healthcare workers are the main experts in the errors, failures, and violations that may exist in their devices. And the solution to these errors can only be offered by technology.

REFERENCES

[1] A. A. Rezaie and A. Habiboghli, "Detection of Lung Nodules on Medical Images by the Use of Fractal Segmentation," *Int. J. Interact. Multimed. Artif. Intell.*, vol. 4, no. 5, 2017.

[2] Y. Ben Youssef et al., "Contour Detection of Mammogram Masses Using ChanVese Model and B-Spline Approximation," *Int. J. Interact. Multimed. Artif. Intell.*, vol. 4, no. 5, 2017.

[3] A. El-Ghobashy, T. Ind, J. Persson, and J. F. Magrina, *Textbook of Gynecologic Robotic Surgery*. Springer, 2018.

[4] Y. P. Kondratenko, P. Khalaf, H. Richter, and D. Simon, "Fuzzy Real-Time Multi-objective Optimization of a Prosthesis Test Robot Control System," in *Advanced Control Techniques in Complex Engineering Systems: Theory and Applications*. Springer, 2019, pp. 165–185.

[5] F. Este, L. Spagna, and G. Bianconi, "Automatic storage and distribution system, and housing unit and picking unit for products packaged in unit doses," *Google Patents*, 2018.

[6] S. Van Buuren, *Flexible Imputation of Missing Data*. Chapman & Hall/CRC, 2018.

[7] D. L. Weed, "Causation: an epidemiologic perspective (in five parts)," *JL Pol'y*, vol. 12, p. 43, 2003.

[8] L. G. Portney et al., *Foundations of Clinical Research: Applications to Practice*, vol. 892. Pearson/Prentice Hall, Upper Saddle River, NJ, 2009.

[9] J. W. Song and K. C. Chung, "Observational studies: cohort and case-control studies," *Plast. Reconstr. Surg.*, vol. 126, no. 6, p. 2234, 2010.

[10] E. Jovanov, A. Lords, D. Raskovic, P. G. Cox, R. Adhami, and F. Andrasik, "Stress monitoring using a distributed wireless intelligent sensor system," *IEEE Eng. Med. Biol. Mag.*, vol. 22, no. 3, pp. 49–55, 2003.

[11] A. Blair et al., "A philosophy for dealing with hypothesized uncontrolled confounding in epidemiological investigations," *Med. DEL Lav.*, vol. 86, p. 106, 1995.
[12] R. P. Singh and M. Dixit, "Histogram equalization: a strong technique for image enhancement," *Int. J. Signal Process. Image Process. Pattern Recognit.*, vol. 8, no. 8, pp. 345–352, 2015.
[13] Z. Yu and C. Bajaj, "A fast and adaptive method for image contrast enhancement," in 2004 International Conference on Image Processing, 2004. ICIP'04., 2004, vol. 2, pp. 1001–1004.
[14] P. K. Saha and J. K. Udupa, "Optimum image thresholding via class uncertainty and region homogeneity," *IEEE Trans. Pattern Anal. Mach. Intell.*, vol. 23, no. 7, pp. 689–706, 2001.
[15] R. Minamimoto et al., "Improvements in PET image quality in time of flight (TOF) simultaneous PET/MRI," *Mol. Imaging Biol.*, vol. 18, no. 5, pp. 776–781, 2016.
[16] S. D. Pathak, D. R. Haynor, and Y. Kim, "Edge-guided boundary delineation in prostate ultrasound images," *IEEE Trans. Med. Imaging*, vol. 19, no. 12, pp. 1211–1219, 2000.
[17] D. L. Pham, C. Xu, and J. L. Prince, "Current methods in medical image segmentation," *Annu. Rev. Biomed. Eng.*, vol. 2, no. 1, pp. 315–337, 2000.
[18] S. Singh, A. Singh, R. Gupta, and S. Sinha, "Automatic Segmentation of Melanoma affected region for Computer-Aided Diagnosis," in 2018 International Conference on Computing, Power and Communication Technologies (GUCON), 2018, pp. 472–475.
[19] C. O. Leong et al., "Segmentation of left ventricle in late gadolinium enhanced MRI through 2D-4D registration for infarct localization in 3D patient-specific left ventricular model," *Magn. Reson. Med.*, vol. 81, no. 2, pp. 1385–1398, 2019.
[20] A. Elgammal and G. Hashing, "CS 534: Computer Vision 3D Model-based recognition," *Dept. Comput. Sci. Rutgers Univ.*, 2004.
[21] INCIBE-CERT. Monitorizando redes y eventos en SCI: más información, más seguridad," INCIBE, 28 Junio 2018. [Online]. Available: https://www.incibe-cert.es/blog/monitorizando-redes-y-eventos-sci-mas-informacion-mas-seguridad. [Accessed April 2019].
[22] Ó. Casas Piedrafita, R. Pallas Areny, and J. Polo Cantero, "Sensórica: el mundo de los sensores y sus interfaces," in *Mundo electrónico. Edición internacional*, no. 410, pp. 34–38, 2010.
[23] J. Muñoz, "La seguridad para Internet de las Cosas en la era del Machine Learning y las Redes Definidas por Software," IoT Futura, 01 Julio 2018. [Online]. Available: https://iotfutura.com/seguridad-iot/seguridad-iot-machine-learning-sdn#Por_que_la_seguridad_IoT_es_tan_complicada. [Accessed April 2019].
[24] M. Khera, "Think like a hacker: Insights on the latest attack vectors (and security controls) for medical device applications," *Journal of Diabetes Science and Technology*, vol. 11, no. 2, pp. 207–212, 2017.
[25] Ley Orgánica 3/2018, de 5 de Diciembre, de Protección de Datos Personales y garantía de los derechos digitales, 2018.
[26] Reglamento (UE) 2016/679 Del Parlamento Europeo y del Consejo relativo a la protección de las personas físicas en lo que respecta al tratamiento de datos personales y a la libre circulación de estos datos y por el que se deroga la Directiva 95/46/CE, 2016.
[27] M. N. Ahmed, A. S. Toor, K. O'Neil and D. Friedland "Cognitive computing and the future of health care cognitive computing and the future of healthcare: the cognitive power of IBM Watson has the potential to transform global personalized medicine," *IEEE Pulse*, vol. 3, no. 8, pp. 4–9, 2017.
[28] Reglamento (CE) 1338/2008 del Parlamento Europeo y del Consejo sobre estadística comunitaria de salud pública y seguridad en el trabajo (DO L 354 de 31.21.2008, p. 70), 2008.

[29] Versión consolidada del Tratado de Funcionamiento de la Unión Europea. Artículo 179 apartado 1, 2012.
[30] E. Aced, "Especial Seguridad y Protección de Datos de Salud," *Sociedad Española de Informática y Salud*, no. 104, pp. 1–50, 2014.
[31] M. Martillo Ramos and J. A. Santamaría Yagual, "Importancia del sistema de seguridad con interconexión para mejorar el bienestar del centro de salud," Universidad de Guayaquil Facultad de Ciencias Administrativas, 2016.
[32] M. Á. A. Moreno, J. B. Gay, J. J. D. Sánchez, F. J. G. López, R. S. Lucena and V. Aguilera, "Seguridad IoT en Sanidad: Estamos Preparados?," Godel Editorial, 2018.

3 An Overview on Wearable Devices for Medical Applications

Meet Kumari[1] *and Meenu Gupta*[2]
[1]Department of Electronics and Communication Engineering, Chandigarh University, Punjab
[2]Department of Computer Science and Engineering, Chandigarh University, Punjab

CONTENTS

3.1 Introduction 37
3.2 Literature Review 38
3.3 Wearable Devices in the Medical Field 40
    3.3.1 Monitoring Used for Wearable Health Devices 41
    3.3.2 Wearable Health Device Technologies for Different Body Parts 41
3.4 Applications 44
3.5 Key Challenges 46
3.6 Conclusion 46
References 46

3.1 INTRODUCTION

In today's world, the interest in wearable computing devices has been increasing because of the potential applications in various fields such as healthcare monitoring of patients. These devices help in observing a patient's vital signs, emergency rescue systems, physical training, etc. [2-4].

As it is well known, lots of diseases could be easily treated if they are detected in an early stage. This leads to saving patients' lives early on. Moreover, the number of people who are 65 years and older is rapidly increasing around the world. This number will double in 2025, i.e., 761 million [5]. Thus, the easiest and most optimal solution to provide the medical facilities is using a low-cost, portable wearable remote monitoring system. However, to identify diseases through a monitoring healthcare application requires medical staff to have crucial information that provides warnings. There is a large interest in researching wearable devices to detect diseases and to provide alarms at an early stage. This helps in maintaining requests and responses among millions of patients through Internet of Things (IoT) [6–8].

Wearable devices for medical applications, or Wearable Health Devices (WHDs), such as sensing and actuating have become the basis of lots of revolutionary digital health fields. Some examples are wearable electrocardiography (ECG) monitors, blood pressure sensors, etc. They consist of sensors, such as motion sensors, which include accelerometers to collect huge amounts of data for medical and fitness applications, record step rate, and monitor acceleration and speed. Also, these sensors can help in collecting information on post-surgery, motor degradation measurement of patients, correlating sleep activity, REM sleep duration, and post-traumatic stress disorders information [9–11].

There are many technologies for power available for WHDs such as resonance-based charging, inductive coupling and microwave. All these are different in terms of working frequency, power level, transfer distance, forming factors and size. All are preferred in different specific applications, such as microwave systems are used over longer distances at low power, inductive coupling systems are used over limited distances at tens of kilowatts, and resonance systems in the megahertz band at tens of watts over tens of centimeter distances. The implantable devices are used over shorter distances; these wireless systems have minimal misalignments. In wristband wearable systems, resonance-based charging systems are most beneficial as compared to others due to their charging distance flexibility and misalignments of sender and receiver coils [12–14].

In this chapter, after presenting an introduction in Section 3.1, Section 3.2 gives a comprehensive literature review. Section 3.3 describes the various wearable devices and their parameters for medical applications. Section 3.4 and 3.5 present the applications and key challenges respectively in wearable devices. Conclusion is drawn in Section 3.6.

3.2 LITERATURE REVIEW

The compact and precise wearable antenna design having a novel Electromagnetic Bandgap (EBG) structure for medical application is presented at 2.4 GHz. It demonstrates a compact, robust and low-profile solution for wearable applications requirements. It is shown that the EBG structure minimizes the effect of frequency detuning and back-radiation because of a large loss of human body. Also, the proposed design antenna having $46 \times 46 \times 2.4$ mm^3 dimension leads to 27% (2.17–2.83 GHz) impedance bandwidth with 7.8 dBi gain. It is concluded that antenna is a potential solution for wearable devices integration in various domains [2].

A human monitoring system is designed and developed to analyze human body ailments. It is shown that smart WHDs may provide people with health data and alerts with various types of sensors, as well as notify them using smartphones. This reduces the load on IoT-connected network and the overall cost of various users. It is also shown that this proposed monitoring system can provide identical communication to various IoT devices [5].

A U-Wear networking framework based on ultrasonic communications for WHDs is presented here. The bit-error-rate achieved (BER) is less than 10^{-5} at 2 kHz bandwidth, 20 mW power and 2.76 kbit/s bit rate. It is concluded that this proposed design can be implemented for reconfigurable data processing applications. It offers higher performance, higher data rates and lower energy consumption [9].

In this chapter, we study the wireless power systems design approach of charging wristband WHDs. This design approach consists of an analytical model that utilizes an optimization algorithm for available wireless power with lateral and angular misalignments. The experimental results confirm the analytical model demonstrates the mutual inductance's performance of the proposed system [12].

The different levels of treatment for medical conditions such as rehabilitation, prevention and immediate care are presented here. Smart textiles or garments have a great impact on treatment, care and prevention of illness. It is possible to integrate the smart garments as a natural step of linking. These garments can provide help to the medical community by giving information about patients' health through remote monitoring. In the future, these garments can provide flexible and adaptable ways for therapeutic functionalities [15].

In this chapter we present a systematic study of security issues in wearable devices. We give a traditional review of the development of security in wearable devices in academia and industry. The adaptive security architecture for preventing adversaries from "breaking through" is discussed to improve the security of architecture layers [16].

We provide a review of wireless WHDs accommodated inside the human body for realizing various stimulating functionalities and sensing. It focuses on in-body medical devices such as those implanted, ingested and injected into the human body. It is concluded that these in-body medical devices are opening up opportunities for prognosis, prevention, as well as treatment far exceeding any design issues of their invasive nature [17].

This chapter shows the latest Wearable Mobile Medical Monitoring Systems (WMMMSs) based on textile and Wireless Sensing Networks (WSNs). These systems consist of different small physiological sensors, processing capabilities and transmission modules. It is concluded that this leads to an effective approach to find the technological merits and demerits of the latest state-of-the-art in WHDs [18].

In this chapter, various improvements of the new wearable technologies are presented in data collection methods in biopharmaceutical research, healthcare, and development. Various applications are identified in many therapeutic areas, facing lots of challenges in scientific methodology, clinical, legal, and operational hurdles and regulation. It is concluded that to further facilitate adoption and evaluation of these technologies for implementation in healthcare areas, we highlight methodological as well as logistical considerations [19].

A state-of the-art review of the wearable sensing platforms for biomedical and healthcare applications is presented here. It has been introduced that stretchable and flexible materials along with sensors help in various emerging wearable physical sensors-based healthcare applications, such as physiological health monitoring, artificial electronic skins, drug delivery and therapeutics [20].

In this chapter, a biometric-based security framework from ECG signals is developed for resource-restrictions wearable medical monitoring and analyzing systems through extracting human heartbeats. The results show that biometric features based on time domain help in optimizing privacy in various IoMT-related healthcare applications. Also, the proposed optimization security model for clinical information provides the validation of the proposed framework utilizing ECG signals from 40 healthy humans. It results in less processing time and less energy. It also provides a trade-off between resource optimization and security [21].

This provides a comprehensive overview of the wearable technology-based applications in terms of safety monitoring. It concludes that the wearable technologies in industrial sectors can be utilized to measure and monitor a large variety of safety metrics in terms of performance in industrial sectors. It also helps in multi-parameter monitoring with the help of wearable sensors for high safety performance [22].

We give here an overview of significant research work on flexible wearable sensors. It is described that these sensors help monitor the physiological parameters, transferring data, etc. Moreover, in the presence of many challenges, these sensors show various future opportunities for different types of applications [23].

We finally review here various WHDs along with their system architectures, specifications and description of the vital signs they acquire. It is concluded that the WHD system presented helps in analyzing commercial devices and their quality versus applicability to extend the subject for medical purposes. Also, the resumed evolution is presented based on developed prototypes. In addition, we describe market trends and challenges of the area of emerging and trending WHDs [24].

The above literature review shows that WHDs are important in daily life and in the future.

3.3 WEARABLE DEVICES IN THE MEDICAL FIELD

WHDs have rapidly increased in various biomedical applications through digital health such as tracking, recording and monitoring. The main aim of these devices is to improve the health of people. The various wearable devices are smart watches, glasses and armbands. The first implantable health device was created in 1960 as a implanted cardiac pacemaker for arrhythmia patients. The Implantable Cardioverter Defibrillators (ICDs) and implantable devices in the deep brain were created to treat millions of patients [25, 26,]. The historical background of various wearable devices is shown in Figure 3.1.

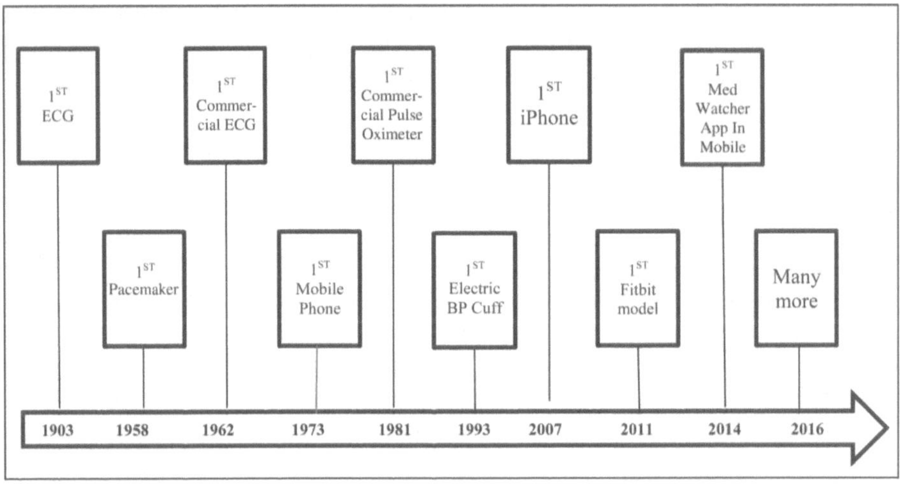

FIGURE 3.1 Historical background of wearable devices for medical applications [19, 27].

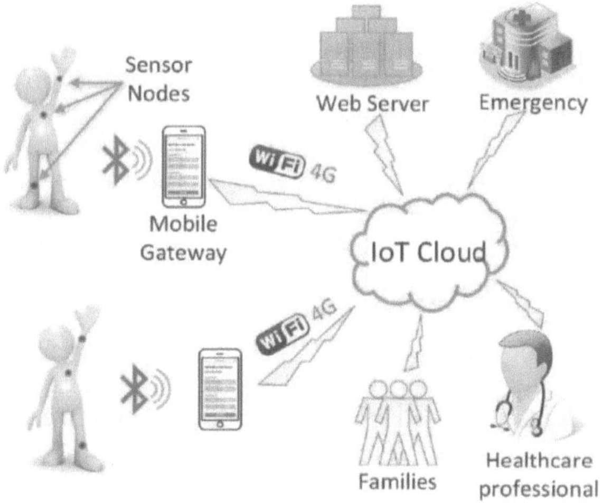

FIGURE 3.2 Wearable health devices for medical applications [30].

3.3.1 Monitoring Used for Wearable Health Devices [28, 29]

Various advanced sensor technologies have been implemented in various wearable sensors and computers used in non-contact or contact mode for healthcare and biomedical applications. Various WHDs are commercially used for regular vital signs monitoring of patients, which is important in modern digital health to allow for transmission of data between a smartphone and the wearable device through Wi-Fi, Bluetooth, etc. These devices help in measuring daily activities of patients, such as calories burned, sleep patterns, step monitoring, eating habits, etc. Others parameters such as blood oxygen saturation level, heart rate, respiration rate, blood pressure, skin temperature, etc. are also monitored through WHDs. Figure 3.2 shows WHDs used for various medical applications [26].

3.3.2 Wearable Health Device Technologies for Different Body Parts

The various WHDs can be worn on various human body parts such as leg/foot, head, or arm, and can be implantable as artificial organs or used as smart pills. The main purpose of these wearable devices is to collect useful health data. Some examples of these WHDs are given as follows [26, 31]:

1. **Head:** This is the uppermost body part and it includes the eyes, nose, forehead and mouth. The WHDs for head are goggles, glasses, contact lenses, headbands, earrings, patches, earphones and hearing aids. The modern smart glasses devices are wearable computers having various sensors, viz., gyroscopes, pressure sensors, image sensors, microphones and accelerometers. Here, voice commands are used for operation by a user interface [26].

2. **Torso:** This central part of the body includes suits, belts, and undershirts worn on the torso. Some examples are pajamas for electrocardiogram measurement in infants, smart jackets for measuring the physiological parameters of babies, uniforms with wearable computers for monitoring military personnel such as UV sensor swimsuits, and glove swaddles of babies for temperature sensing. These can used for continuous monitoring and enhancing patient health. Moreover, a plaster for sweat analysis, pain relief, repelling mosquitoes and patches for drug delivery are also demonstrated. In addition, smart bras, shirts and a wearable artificial pancreas are some of the examples [26, 32].
3. **Arm, foot and leg:** Here, the WHDs worn on the arm, foot and leg such as bracelets, smartwatches, armbands, wristbands, rings, etc. to monitor physiological parameters like body temperature, heart rate, daily activities and UV exposure levels. This also includes smartsocks, sleeves and other wearable accessories worn on the leg or foot [26, 32]. Various wireless technologies and privacy controls for wearable devices in medical applications are shown in Table 3.1 and Table 3.2 [9,34].

The commercial WHDs and their sensors are shown in Table 3.3.

TABLE 3.1
Wireless Communication Technologies Used for Wearable Devices [19,26,35]

Wireless Communication-Technology	Standard	Frequency (GHz)	Distance (m)	Data Rate (Mbps)	Modulation	Power (mW)	Summary
Bluetooth	IEEE802.15.1	2.4	10	1	FHSS	100	Fast, high mobility and high power consumption
ZigBee	IEEE802.15.4	0.8–2.4	75	20–250	DSSS	<100	Low cost, less power, large network, safe and reliable
NFC	IEC18092	0.013	0.02	106–424	ASK	<100	Small range, security required
UWB	IEEE802.15.3	3.1–10.6	>100	100–1024	OFDM	<=1	Wide bandwidth, confidentialand less transmission power
Wi-Fi	IEEE802.11a/b/g	2.4	<100	11	OFDM and DSSS	70	Fast transmission and high power consumption

Note: ASK: Amplitude Shift Keying, DSSS: Direct Sequence Spread Spectrum, FHSS: Frequency Hopping Spread Spectrum, NFC: Near Field Communication, OFDM: Orthogonal Frequency Division Multiplexing, UWB: Ultra Wideband.

TABLE 3.2
Families of Privacy Controls in Wearable Health Devices [19,36]

No.	Control Family	Examples
1	Access Control	Access Enforcement, Account Management and Information Flow Enforcement
2	Audit and Accountability	Audit Management Event, Reporting and Analysis of Audit Review
3	Awareness and Training	Role-based Training and General Awareness Training
4	Assessment, Authorization and Monitoring	Assessment Guidelines, Annual Assessments and Independent Assessment
5	Contingency Planning	Contingency Training, Contingency Plan and Testing Contingency Plan
6	Configuration Management	Configuration Change Control and Baseline Configuration
7	Identification, Authentication	Device Management, User Management and Management of Specific Identifiers
8	Incident Response	Training, Incident Response Rules and Policies, Monitoring, Procedures and Handling
9	Individual Participation	Redress, ACT Statements, Individual Consent and Access
10	Media Protection	Media Marking, Sanitization and Use, Media Access and Storage, and Transport
11	Maintenance	Maintenance Tools, Controlled Maintenance Local and Non-local
12	Physical and Environmental Protection	Monitoring, Control and Physical Access Authorization
13	Privacy Authorization	Purpose and Sharing and Authority to Collect
14	Planning	Updates, Impact Assessments, Security and Privacy Plans and Rules of Behavior
15	Personnel Security	Risk Designation, Personnel Screening and Transfer and Termination
16	Program Management	Roles, Resources, Program Plan, Architecture and Performance and Inventory
17	Risk Assessment	Vulnerability and Assessment Scanning, Security Categorization
18	System and Telecommunication Protection	Security Isolation Function, Application Partitioning and Boundary security and Protection
19	System, Services Acquisition	Documentation, Systems Lifecycle, Resource Allocation and Acquisition
20	Information Integrity	Malicious Code Protection, Alerts and Advisories, Flaw Remediation and Monitoring

TABLE 3.3
Commercial Wearable Health Devices and Their Sensors [26,36,37]

No.	Vital Sign	Wearable Health Device	Sensor
1	Heart rate	Ear-O-Smart, Cosinuss One earpiece, Bragi, Samsung Gear Fit, Basis, Go2 Fingertip Pulse Oximeter, Avery Dennison Metria, Phyode W/Me Wristband, iHealth, Omron, Google Glass, PoloTech	Pulse oximeter, electrocardiogram, pressure, gyroscope, accelerometer, image, 3D accelerometer
2	Blood oxygen saturation	Bragi, Go2 Fingertip Pulse Oximeter	Pulse oximeter
3	Body and/or skin temperature	Cosinuss One earpiece, Bragi, Basis	Temperature
4	Respiration rate	Spire, Smart textile electrocardiogram, Glass	Accelerometer, piezo-resistive, gyroscope, accelerometer, image
5	Blood pressure	Sensor, Patch, iHealth, Omron	Potential difference, pressure, photoplethysmography

3.4 APPLICATIONS

The various potential applications of WHDs are shown as follows:

1. **Adaptive care provisioning:** Artificial Intelligence (AI) and Machine Learning (ML) based healthcare applications play an important role in revolutionalizing the healthcare system by focusing on adaptive and automatic care provisioning. Various intelligent and statistical models are developed for presenting non-linear and linear models for neural networks [21,38,39].
2. **Remote healthcare monitoring:** The WHD related to health monitoring systems provides the feature sharing and connection capability with wireless devices technologies for various continuous and discrete event management. It includes various platforms such as military operations, farms, fields, theaters, etc. [4].
3. **Stroke restoration:** This can be used for video conferencing featuring transmission of medical information to various remote areas, thus increasing the effectiveness, level of tele-rehabilitation recognition and viability for stroke victims [21,40,41].
4. **Wireless portable capsule endoscopy:** This is a part of tele-healthcare and tele-monitoring for vital sign users in a medical market. This is imperative to send all medical data like physiological signals, image signals and video. It is one of the paradigms in the medical market that provide patients and physicians commercial capabilities [21,42,43].

TABLE 3.4
Applications of Wearable Health Devices through Various Wireless Technologies [9,45,46]

No.	Application	NFC Enabled Platform
1	Health monitoring such as ECG, bio-signals and SpO_2	Smartphone-based terminal
2	Monitoring and identification of patients in clinics or hospitals	Server, reader device and identification
3	BP, temperature, body weight, HR, C-reactive protein, etc.	Smartphone-based terminal
4	Remote monitoring	Smartphone-based terminal
5	Tele-monitoring	Smartphone-based terminal
6	Fetal health monitoring	Smartphone-based terminal
7	Heart rate monitoring	Smartphone-based terminal

5. **Emergency medical healthcare:** The main goal of this application is to facilitate for doctors and patients the efficient medical care of cardiovascular diseases, especially, for emergency patients. Thus, there is a need for intelligent and smart sensor-based devices for managing the whole process as well as the mechanism of a patient's medical care [21,44]. Also, others potential applications of WHDs are shown in Table 3.4 and Table 3.5.

TABLE 3.5
Some Wearable Health Devices for Medical Applications [19,47]

No.	Wearable Device	Collected Data	Examples
1	Wrist-wearing device	Actigraphy, HR, BP, EDA	ActiGraph Link through ActiGraph, Actiwatch Spectrum through Phillips, E4 by Empatica, ViSi Mobile through Sotera Wireless
2	Cuffs	BP, HR	Intellisense Digital BP Monitoring
3	Headbands	EEG, EMG	4D FORCE through 4D FORCE EMOTIV EPOC through Emotiv
4	Skin patch	Skin temperature, ECG, actigraphy	BioStampRC by MC10 BodyGuardian through Preventice HealthPatch through Vital Connect
5	Finger-wearing device	HR, SpO_2	iSpO_2 Pulse Oximeter through Massimo
6	Sensors used in clothes	HR, HRV, breathing rate, ECG, actigraphy	Innovative shirts through Hexoskin

3.5 KEY CHALLENGES

Successful WHD development may enable the large applications ranging from single-person healthcare to multiple persons. All of these applications have many security concerns and challenges. Here, some major concerns and challenges are discussed for the various WHD applications as follows [16, 48, 49]:

1. **Information confidentiality:** In WHDs, healthcare data should be confidential. In current healthcare monitoring systems, various WHDs forward and accumulate medical information to a central location. A hacker can spy on this information. This leads to various challenges to the affected patients, as hackers may utilize the accumulated and sensitive medical information for illegal purposes [21, 50, 51].
2. **Information integrity:** The confidentiality and integrity of healthcare data is a major factor for the WHD transmission. Hackers can modify the medical information by introducing fake fragments within the real data and delivering it to the receiver node. Ensuring data integrity is the prominent solution from external attacks [21, 52].
3. **Information availability:** In terms of WHDs, it is very important that medical data and system resources information be accessible to all users [21, 53].

3.6 CONCLUSION

In this chapter, various Wearable Health Devices (WHDs) for medical applications have been discussed. It is concluded these devices are inseparable part of our digital modern life today. Various researchers are working on improving these devices and to promote them in order to help more and more people of all ages. Also, although these devices face various challenges, their application in the present and future makes them more attractive among doctors, patients and everyday persons.

REFERENCES

[1] Nguyen, C. T., "Enabling and Emerging Technologies for Social Distancing: A Comprehensive Survey and Open Problems", *arXiv e-prints*, 2020.

[2] Ashyap, A. Y. I.; Zainal Abidin, Z.; Dahlan, S. H.; Majid, H. A.; Shah, S. M.; Kamarudin, M. R.; Alomainy, A.; Compact and Low-Profile Textile EBG-Based Antenna for Wearable Medical Applications. *IEEE Antennas Wirel. Propag. Lett.*, 2017, *16* (July), 2550–2553. https://doi.org/10.1109/LAWP.2017.2732355.

[3] Cuartero, M.; Parrilla, M.; Crespo, G. A.; Wearable Potentiometric Sensors for Medical Applications. *Sensors (Switzerland)*, 2019, *19* (2), 1–24. https://doi.org/10.3390/s19020363.

[4] Clarke, R.; What Drones Inherit from Their Ancestors. *Comput. Law Secur. Rev.*, 2014, *30* (3), 247–262. https://doi.org/10.1016/j.clsr.2014.03.006.

[5] United Nations, Department of Economic and Social Affairs Population Division, World Population Ageing 2015. New York, 2015.

[6] Nassar, A.; A Survey on Smart Cities IoT (Internet of Things). *Proc. Int. Conf. Adv. Intell. Syst. Informatics*, 2018, *639* (1), 1–10. https://doi.org/10.1007/978-3-319-64861-3.

[7] Georgiou, K.; Larentzakis, A. V.; Khamis, N. N.; Alsuhaibani, G. I.; Alaska, Y. A.; Giallafos, E. J.; Can Wearable Devices Accurately Measure Heart Rate Variability? A Systematic Review. *Folia Med. (Plovdiv).*, 2018, *60* (1), 7–20. https://doi.org/10.2478/folmed-2018-0012.

[8] Warkentin, M.; Orgeron, C.; Using the Security Triad to Assess Blockchain Technology in Public Sector Applications. *Int. J. Inf. Manage.*, 2020, 102090. https://doi.org/10.1016/j.ijinfomgt.2020.102090.

[9] Ding, G.; Wu, Q.; Zhang, L.; Lin, Y.; Tsiftsis, T. A.; Yao, Y. D.; An Amateur Drone Surveillance System Based on the Cognitive Internet of Things. *IEEE Commun. Mag.*, 2018, *56* (1), 29–35. https://doi.org/10.1109/MCOM.2017.1700452.

[10] Santagati, G. E.; Melodia, T.; A Software-Defined Ultrasonic Networking Framework for Wearable Devices. *IEEE/ACM Trans. Netw.*, 2017, *25* (2), 960–973. https://doi.org/10.1109/TNET.2016.2616724.

[11] Szydło, T.; Konieczny, M.; Mobile and Wearable Devices in an Open and Universal System for Remote Patient Monitoring. *Microprocess. Microsyst.*, 2016, *46*, 44–54. https://doi.org/10.1016/j.micpro.2016.07.006.

[12] Makhdoom, I.; Abolhasan, M.; Abbas, H.; Ni, W.; Blockchain's Adoption in IoT: The Challenges, and a Way Forward. *J. Netw. Comput. Appl.*, 2019, *125*, 251–279. https://doi.org/10.1016/j.jnca.2018.10.019.

[13] Roshan, Y. M.; Park, E. J.; Design Approach for a Wireless Power Transfer System for Wristband Wearable Devices. *IET Power Electron.*, 2017, *10* (8), 931–937. https://doi.org/10.1049/iet-pel.2016.0616.

[14] Cheng, J. W.; Mitomo, H.; The Underlying Factors of the Perceived Usefulness of Using Smart Wearable Devices for Disaster Applications. *Telemat. Informatics*, 2017, *34* (2), 528–539. https://doi.org/10.1016/j.tele.2016.09.010.

[15] Si, H.; Sun, C.; Li, Y.; Qiao, H.; Shi, L.; IoT Information Sharing Security Mechanism Based on Blockchain Technology. *Futur. Gener. Comput. Syst.*, 2019, *101*, 1028–1040. https://doi.org/10.1016/j.future.2019.07.036.

[16] Coyle, S.; Diamond, D.; Medical Applications of Smart Textiles. In *Advances in Smart Medical Textiles: Treatments and Health Monitoring*; 2016; pp. 215–237. https://doi.org/10.1016/B978-1-78242-379-9.00010-4.

[17] Wang, S.; Bie, R.; Zhao, F.; Zhang, N.; Cheng, X.; Choi, H. A.; Security in Wearable Communications. *IEEE Netw.*, 2016, *30* (5), 61–67. https://doi.org/10.1109/MNET.2016.7579028.

[18] Kiourti, A.; Nikita, K. S.; A Review of In-Body Biotelemetry Devices: Implantables, Ingestibles, and Injectables. *IEEE Trans. Biomed. Eng.*, 2017, *64* (7), 1422–1430. https://doi.org/10.1109/TBME.2017.2668612.

[19] Liang, T.; Yuan, Y. J.; Wearable Medical Monitoring Systems Based on Wireless Networks: A Review. *IEEE Sens. J.*, 2016, *16* (23), 8186–8199. https://doi.org/10.1109/JSEN.2016.2597312.

[20] Izmailova, E. S.; Wagner, J. A.; Perakslis, E. D.; Wearable Devices in Clinical Trials: Hype and Hypothesis. *Clin. Pharmacol. Ther.*, 2018, *104* (1), 42–52. https://doi.org/10.1002/cpt.966.

[21] Kenry; Yeo, J. C.; Lim, C. T.; Emerging Flexible and Wearable Physical Sensing Platforms for Healthcare and Biomedical Applications. *Microsystems Nanoeng.*, 2016, *2* (April). 119. https://doi.org/10.1038/micronano.2016.43.

[22] Pirbhulal, S.; Samuel, O. W.; Wu, W.; Sangaiah, A. K.; Li, G.; A Joint Resource-Aware and Medical Data Security Framework for Wearable Healthcare Systems. *Futur. Gener. Comput. Syst.*, 2019, *95* (January), 382–391. https://doi.org/10.1016/j.future.2019.01.008.

[23] Awolusi, I.; Marks, E.; Hallowell, M.; Wearable Technology for Personalized Construction Safety Monitoring and Trending: Review of Applicable Devices. *Autom. Constr.*, 2018, *85* (October 2017), 96–106. https://doi.org/10.1016/j.autcon.2017.10.010.

[24] Nag, A.; Mukhopadhyay, S. C.; Kosel, J.; Wearable Flexible Sensors: A Review. *IEEE Sens. J.*, 2017, *17* (13), 3949–3960. https://doi.org/10.1109/JSEN.2017.2705700.
[25] Dias, D.; Cunha, J. P. S.; Wearable Health Devices—Vital Sign Monitoring, Systems and Technologies. *Sensors (Switzerland)*, 2018, *18* (8). https://doi.org/10.3390/s18082414.
[26] Mistry, I.; Tanwar, S.; Tyagi, S.; Kumar, N.; Blockchain for 5G-Enabled IoT for Industrial Automation : A Systematic Review, Solutions, and Challenges. *Mech. Syst. Signal Process.*, 2020, *135*, 106382. https://doi.org/10.1016/j.ymssp.2019.106382.
[27] Rishani, N.; Elayan, H.; Shubair, R.; Kiourti, A.; Wearable, Epidermal, and Implantable Sensors for Medical Applications. *arXiv*:1810.00321, 2018, 1–20.
[28] Spagnolli, A.; Guardigli, E.; Orso, V.; Varotto, A.; Gamberini, L.; Measuring User Acceptance of Wearable Symbiotic Devices: Validation Study across Application Scenarios. *Lect. Notes Comput. Sci. (including Subser. Lect. Notes Artif. Intell. Lect. Notes Bioinformatics)*, 2014, *8820*, 87–98. https://doi.org/10.1007/978-3-319-13500-7_7.
[29] King, R. C.; Villeneuve, E.; White, R. J.; Sherratt, R. S.; Holderbaum, W.; Harwin, W. S.; Application of Data Fusion Techniques and Technologies for Wearable Health Monitoring. *Med. Eng. Phys.*, 2017, *42*, 1–12. https://doi.org/10.1016/j.medengphy.2016.12.011.
[30] Sodhro, A. H.; Pirbhulal, S.; Sangaiah, A. K.; Convergence of IoT and Product Lifecycle Management in Medical Health Care. *Futur. Gener. Comput. Syst.*, 2018, *86* (April), 380–391. https://doi.org/10.1016/j.future.2018.03.052.
[31] Wu, T.; Wu, F.; Redoute, J. M.; Yuce, M. R.; An Autonomous Wireless Body Area Network Implementation Towards IoT Connected Healthcare Applications. *IEEE Access*, 2017, *5*, 11413–11422. https://doi.org/10.1109/ACCESS.2017.2716344.
[32] Banos, O.; Garcia, R.; Holgado-terriza, J. A.; Damas, M.; MHealthDroid: A Novel Framework for Agile Development of Mobile Health Applications Oresti. *International Workshop on Ambient Assisted Living*, 2014, *8868* (March 2015), 90–98. https://doi.org/10.1007/978-3-319-13105-4.
[33] Bera, B.; Chattaraj, D.; Das, A. K.; Designing Secure Blockchain-Based Access Control Scheme in IoT-Enabled Internet of Drones Deployment. *Comput. Commun.*, 2020, *153*, 229–249. https://doi.org/10.1016/j.comcom.2020.02.011.
[34] Jawad, S. S.; Fyath, R. S.; Transmission Performance of Analog Radio-over-Fiber Fronthaul for 5G Mobile Networks. *International Journal of Networks and Communications*, 2018, *8* (3), 81–96. https://doi.org/10.5923/j.ijnc.20180803.03.
[35] Sodhro, A. H.; Sangaiah, A. K.; Pirphulal, S.; Sekhari, A.; Ouzrout, Y.; Green Media-Aware Medical IoT System. *Multimed. Tools Appl.*, 2019, *78* (3), 3045–3064. https://doi.org/10.1007/s11042-018-5634-0.
[36] Chávez-Santiago, R.; Khaleghi, A.; Balasingham, I.; Ramstad, T. A.; Architecture of an Ultra Wideband Wireless Body Area Network for Medical Applications. *2nd Int. Symp. Appl. Sci. Biomed. Commun. Technol. ISABEL 2009*, 2009, https://doi.org/10.1109/ISABEL.2009.5373624.
[37] Amjadi, M.; Kyung, K. U.; Park, I.; Sitti, M.; Stretchable, Skin-Mountable, and Wearable Strain Sensors and Their Potential Applications: A Review. *Adv. Funct. Mater.*, 2016, *26* (11), 1678–1698. https://doi.org/10.1002/adfm.201504755.
[38] Preuveneers, D.; Joosen, W.; Privacy-Enabled Remote Health Monitoring Applications for Resource Constrained Wearable Devices. *Proc. ACM Symp. Appl. Comput.*, 2016, *04-08-April*, 119–124. https://doi.org/10.1145/2851613.2851683.
[39] Mundt, C. W.; Montgomery, K. N.; Udoh, U. E.; Barker, V. N.; Thonier, G. C.; Tellier, A. M.; Ricks, R. D.; Darling, R. B.; Cagle, Y. D.; Cabrol, N. A.; et al.; A Multiparameter Wearable Physiologic Monitoring System for Space and Terrestrial Applications. *IEEE Trans. Inf. Technol. Biomed.*, 2005, *9* (3), 382–391. https://doi.org/10.1109/TITB.2005.854509.

[40] Pereira, A. A.; Espada, J. P.; Crespo, R. G.; Aguilar, S. R.; Platform for Controlling and Getting Data from Network Connected Drones in Indoor Environments. *Futur. Gener. Comput. Syst.*, 2019, *92*, 656–662. https://doi.org/10.1016/j.future.2018.01.011.
[41] Teng, X. F.; Poon, C. C. Y.; Zhang, Y. T.; Bonato, P.; Wearable Medical Systems for P-Health. *IEEE Rev. Biomed. Eng.*, 2008, *1* (February), 62–74. https://doi.org/10.1109/RBME.2008.2008248.
[42] Mukherjee, A.; Dey, N.; De, D.; EdgeDrone: QoS Aware MQTT Middleware for Mobile Edge Computing in Opportunistic Internet of Drone Things. *Comput. Commun.*, 2020, *152* (January), 93–108. https://doi.org/10.1016/j.comcom.2020.01.039.
[43] Lukowicz, P.; Lukowicz, P.; Kirstein, T.; Tröster, G.; L11 - Wearable Systems for Health Care Applications. *Methods Inf. Med.*, 2014, *43* (July), 232–238. https://doi.org/10.1267/METH04030232.
[44] Knieps, G.; Internet of Things, Big Data and the Economics of Networked Vehicles. *Telecomm. Policy*, 2019, *43* (2), 171–181. https://doi.org/10.1016/j.telpol.2018.09.002.
[45] De La Torre, G.; Rad, P.; Choo, K. K. R.; Driverless Vehicle Security: Challenges and Future Research Opportunities. *Futur. Gener. Comput. Syst.*, 2018. https://doi.org/10.1016/j.future.2017.12.041.
[46] Berglund, M. E.; Duvall, J.; Dunne, L. E.; A Survey of the Historical Scope and Current Trends of Wearable Technology Applications. *Int. Symp. Wearable Comput. Dig. Pap.*, 2016, *12-16-Sept.*, 40–43. https://doi.org/10.1145/2971763.2971796.
[47] Moin, S.; Karim, A.; Safdar, Z.; Safdar, K.; Ahmed, E.; Imran, M.; Securing IoTs in Distributed Blockchain : Analysis, Requirements and Open Issues. *Futur. Gener. Comput. Syst.*, 2019, *100*, 325–343. https://doi.org/10.1016/j.future.2019.05.023.
[48] Zavitsanou, S.; Chakrabarty, A.; Dassau, E.; Doyle, F. J.; Embedded Control in Wearable Medical Devices: Application to the Artificial Pancreas. *Processes*, 2016, *4* (4).1–29 https://doi.org/10.3390/pr4040035.
[49] Alrige M., Chatterjee S. (2015) Toward a Taxonomy of Wearable Technologies in Healthcare. In: Donnellan B., Helfert M., Kenneally J., VanderMeer D., Rothenberger M., Winter R. (eds) *New Horizons in Design Science: Broadening the Research Agenda. DESRIST 2015. Lecture Notes in Computer Science*, 496–504, vol 9073. Springer, Cham. https://doi.org/10.1007/978-3-319-18714-3_43
[50] Sengupta, J.; Ruj, S.; Das, S.; Journal of Network and Computer Applications A Comprehensive Survey on Attacks, Security Issues and Blockchain Solutions for IoT and IIoT. *J. Netw. Comput. Appl.*, 2020, *149* (April 2019), 102481. https://doi.org/10.1016/j.jnca.2019.102481.
[51] Tian, Y.; Yuan, J.; Song, H.; Efficient Privacy-Preserving Authentication Framework for Edge-Assisted Internet of Drones. *J. Inf. Secur. Appl.*, 2019, *48*, 102354. https://doi.org/10.1016/j.jisa.2019.06.010.
[52] Yaqoob, I.; Ahmed, E.; Rehman, M. H.; Ahmed, A. I. A.; Al-garadi, M. A.; Imran, M.; Guizani, M.; The Rise of Ransomware and Emerging Security Challenges in the Internet of Things. *Comput. Networks*, 2017, *129*, 444–458. https://doi.org/10.1016/j.comnet.2017.09.003.
[53] Sicari, S.; Rizzardi, A.; Grieco, L. A.; Coen-Porisini, A.; Security, Privacy and Trust in Internet of Things: The Road Ahead. *Comput. Networks*, 2015, *76*, 146–164. https://doi.org/10.1016/j.comnet.2014.11.008.
[54] Renduchintala, A.; Jahan, F.; Khanna, R.; Javaid, A. Y.; A Comprehensive Micro Unmanned Aerial Vehicle (UAV/Drone) Forensic Framework. *Digit. Investig.*, 2019, *30* (2019), 52–72. https://doi.org/10.1016/j.diin.2019.07.002.

4 Blockchain-Based IoT for Personalized Pharmaceuticals

Rehab A. Rayan[1] *and Christos Tsagkaris*[2]
[1]Department of Epidemiology, High Institute of Public Health, Alexandria University, Egypt.
[2]Faculty of Medicine, University of Crete, Heraklion, Greece.

CONTENTS

4.1 Introduction 51
4.2 Blockchain Technology in Healthcare 52
4.3 The Internet of Things in Healthcare 53
4.4 Applications of the IoT and Blockchain in the Pharmaceutical Industry 54
 4.4.1 The Smart Fridge 54
 4.4.2 Promoting Virtual Clinical Trials 55
 4.4.3 Fighting Fake Medications 55
 4.4.4 Enhancing 3-D Printing of Medications 56
 4.4.5 Cryptopharmaceuticals 57
4.5 Discussions 58
4.6 Limitations 58
4.7 Conclusions 59
References 59

4.1 INTRODUCTION

Recently, the pharmaceutical industry is faced with the need for changing the design of drug products. Upcoming medications shall possess novel characteristics, such as intrinsic personalized components coupled with information and tracking aspects. Late advances in the genetics discipline opened a window to account for more personalized and customized management approaches. Mapping genes offers information for predicting health risks, and hence advancing management approaches. Genomic medicine has been deployed in some marketed monoclonal antibody cancer therapies [1]. Meanwhile, growing advances in diagnostic point-of-care sensors made it possible to measure respiration, temperature, biomarkers from sweat, and emotions via the modern wearable sensors embedded into clothes [2]. Such health-related facets from the view of the IoT would produce a novel form of human–machine interaction regarding therapies [3]. However, the produced solutions for current dosage forms are challenging to be incorporated into the forthcoming IoT-derived health model [4].

The current health model needs to be enhanced, to optimize personalized medicine, in all aspects from finding novel drug products to communicating with the consumer (patient). Delivering individualized care necessitates a breakthrough in the health domain and a drastic modification in designing, producing, and distributing personalized drug products. The existing fixed-dose pattern of mass-production for medicinal products does not offer adjusting or personalization of medicine according to personal genes, metabolism, or the level of activity. Hence, the concepts of pharmaceutical product design should be shifted toward the mass adaptation of information-based medicinal products [5]. The process of pharmaceutical product discovery and development needs improvement via enrolling patients in patient-centered clinical trials and applying the principle of the digitalized patient into the needed data handling framework, while adhering to the existing data safeguard standards with no breaching of patient safety. Such a principle covers the domain of Big Data and machine learning-driven diagnosis [6–8].

Nowadays, investing in the pharmaceutical industry is generally devoted to finding drugs and, usually, the resulting product is designed applying legacy guidelines; for example, the ancient compaction technique for designing solid dosage forms (tablets) [9]. Ultimately, the production process is usually conventional and unwilling to change, primarily for the associated legislative and reporting workload [10, 11]. Yet, the gross medication prices have risen drastically, adding to the fiscal burden of the community and hitting unsatisfactory levels. Hence, a novel technique is highly needed to minimize the medication cost via reconsidering the drug product design guidelines, associated production interventions, and distribution patterns. Such a technique would secure access to affordable, safe, and effective medicines by switching from the batch manufacturing of fixed-dose products to producing on-demand individualized products. Such products could be designed to include information-rich models; for instance, rapid responding codes, facilitating monitoring of a single product from the production unit to the patient side [12].

4.2 BLOCKCHAIN TECHNOLOGY IN HEALTHCARE

Blockchain stands for a computational system capable of recording transactions conducted in cryptocurrency and maintaining them across several computers interconnected in a peer-to-peer network [13]. Although its origin can be traced back to finance and transactions, in the previous years, its use has been extrapolated to other fields because of its inherent features and of the transaction-based model of operation that these fields have incorporated. As far as its inherent features are concerned, blockchain comprises various features including distributed ledger, decentralized storage, authentication, security, and immutability. As far as the spread of a transaction-based operational model across disciplines is concerned, healthcare services in terms of insurance are considered as providers delivering care as a product. These transactions include an impressive deal of personal, confidential, and technical data with potential implications on individuals' well-being and professional development, among others [14]. Violations of such data have led many voices to support a blockchain healthcare provision system, where practitioners will gain more autonomy, and patients will not be afraid of having their data communicated with third parties [15].

Except for doctor–patient communication and individual patient records, other elements of healthcare need similar technical infrastructure. The pharmaceutical sector is probably one of the most crucial. A popular saying goes like, "All drugs can be a poison; the dosage makes them either remedy or poison". Amid the 4th Industrial Revolution, this quote could be recited in terms of pharmaceutical data [16]. There is a huge data flow concerning medicines, not only those that are already in use, but especially those that are currently developed and tested. Clinical trials, the process of testing novel medicines on humans, is based on the quality and the quantity of data testifying for the efficacy and the safety of an agent compared to a placebo. Any information related to the participants is to remain confidential by law. Most times, even researchers ought not to link participants' identities with individual outcomes for the sake of randomization [17]. Emerging branches of pharmaceutical science, particularly pharmacovigilance and pharmacogenomics, require a significant amount of data to be safely stored and processed. Unauthorized access to such information can lead to falsified approval and allegation on medicines menacing not only doctor–patient communication, but also the life and well-being of patients [18].

Why can blockchain contribute to this need? The biomedical applications of blockchain require more stringent authentication, interoperability, and record sharing modalities. These requirements stand on ethical and legal grounds, taking into account the Health Insurance Portability and Accountability Act of 1996 (HIPAA) and the General Data Protection Regulation of 2018 (GDPR) [14, 19]. Adapting existing blockchain modalities to the context of healthcare has already led to considerable advances and generated even more hope. Such modalities include smart contracts, fraud detection, and sound systems of identification. In pharmaceuticals, all the aforementioned can work as additional valves safeguarding integrity and confidentiality and subsequently producing reliable data. There are still concerns regarding the inherent vulnerabilities of blockchain and the inadequate digital literacy of the users, let alone mining incentives, attacks, and key management [20].

4.3 THE INTERNET OF THINGS IN HEALTHCARE

The Internet of Things (IoT) is described as a network of physical devices that uses connectivity to enable the exchange of data. These devices can either be conventional contemporary or cutting-edge technology. What is remarkable about the IoT is the fast streamline processes that enable workers to complete given tasks in a timely way. The IoT is expected to be supported by the 5G network infrastructure, which guarantees the speed of large datasets' transfer and analysis [21]. In the last years, public or private entities specialized in healthcare or technology have directed their interest and investment in the IoT. Nowadays, most of the existing devices, from smartphones with health-related apps to wearable biosensors and imaging machines, are manufactured with connectivity modalities such as infrared, Bluetooth, or Wireless Fidelity (Wi-Fi). This is a remarkable asset to form data-exchange networks where the provision of healthcare relies on the exchange of data, such as imaging and laboratory tests, patient records, and research results [21, 22].

IoT-enabled medical devices provide critical data transfer and analysis services that assist healthcare practitioners and researchers in a wide range of tasks, from emergency to regular procedures. The benefit of incorporating IoT modalities in healthcare is twofold. Not only it facilitates a large load of work to improve and speed up biomedical research and clinical practice, but it also relieves some burden of health practitioners allowing them to be more creative and more empathetic [14, 23]. The potential impact of the IoT infrastructure in remote patient monitoring, treatment progress, and outcome observation, vaccines, and medicines research has become obvious. In terms of cost, any similar IoT health platform can be owned and operated by a specialized center, providing services to patients all over a region or even a country. So far there have been a few IoT applications in healthcare finding their way to clinical practice [24].

Beyond the collection and analysis of data, IoT data analysis platforms such as Kaa (KaaIoT Technologies), MindSphere (Siemens) and Azure (Microsoft) have IoT-based data processing features leading to meaningful actionable trends. Such modalities are expected to be used widely as far as commercial fitness and biosensors are concerned. Physical activity levels in combination with caloric burn and intake, nutritional and medicines compliance data and blood pressure, heart rate, and blood glucose monitoring have already been valuable at an individual level and can make a difference if extrapolated in population research by IoT modalities. Human control is also important, but if the collection and processing are semi-automated, or even automated, it can speed up the production of the results and their translation in clinical practice [25, 26].

4.4 APPLICATIONS OF THE IoT AND BLOCKCHAIN IN THE PHARMACEUTICAL INDUSTRY

As previously mentioned, blockchain is a developing set of ledgers (chunks) where the ledgers are linked together by the hashing cryptographic technology. The highly famous application of this technology is the cryptocurrency bitcoin. An effort of large-scale blockchain integration in healthcare is currently taking place in countries like the United Kingdom. Starting from January 2016, the authorities have communicated relevant information. This stated the National Health Service as a potential beneficiary of blockchain modalities, to improve authentic delivery of services and communicating patients' records and sensitive information in a confidential and secure manner, abiding by the existing regulations [27]. Philips with the Philips Blockchain Lab has partnered with blockchain record-keeping start-up Tierion to examine how blockchain technology could be used in the healthcare sector since 2018 [27]. Regarding the pharmaceutical setting, blockchain implies interesting potential such as investigating a lifelong medication history.

4.4.1 THE SMART FRIDGE

The Smart Fridge for vaccines by Weka is an interesting example of IoT in health. It addresses mainstay issues in vaccine management and storing such as maintaining the recommended temperature, ensuring the provision of stable electrical current, and tackling other inventory errors resulting in spoilage. The Weka Smart Fridge allows remote monitoring to ensure vaccines are stored at the correct temperature and automated inventory management services allow clinicians to feel at ease and updated about storing vaccines [28]. It is accompanied by a kiosk allowing practitioners to schedule the use of vaccines, making single vials accessible instead of exposing the whole content to environmental conditions. Overall, the Smart Fridge is an IoT modality capable of streamlining the handling of vaccines. Secondary analysis of data by large-scale use of such fridges can evaluate trends regarding the compliance of practitioners to vaccination programs [28, 29].

4.4.2 Promoting Virtual Clinical Trials

Clinical trials, a critical issue in the drug industry, are burdensome and costly sections in developing novel medicines. Such rising expenses are because of the challenges in finding and enrolling competent individuals, organizing and controlling personalized procedures for many subjects over a long time, and dealing with the rising levels of loss-to-follow-up. Organizing personalized procedures is costly for the demand to enroll individuals from definite areas, having access to special clinical trial centers, and to recruit dedicated and competent clinical personnel. The regional limits restrict the patterns and numbers of the trial sample [30].

Virtual clinical trials could diversify the sample, deliver a personalized experience, and minimize requiring dedicated clinical personnel. The drug industry has adopted virtual techniques, especially with non-interventional clinical trials, and achieved variable outcomes for many factors involving the accuracy, protection, and confidentially of data and problems of credibility, regulated adherence, and managing consents. The blockchain technique combined with the IoT-integrated sensors and wearables could enable adequate credibility, protection, and confidentiality of data as demanded by regulating bodies [31].

Blockchain technologies enable an intelligent technique of contracting to guarantee instantly that the participants' consent information is recorded, electronically signed, and sufficiently accountable. The incentives offered to the trial individuals would be token-based, instead of the present-date money-based ones, for growing participation, enhancing adherence, and developing more personalized experience. Finding and enrolling the trial individuals could be considerably simplified if the archived clinical data were accessible via a blockchain-derived Personalized Health Record (PHR), assuring beneficiaries that their data would be safeguarded devoid jeopardizing privacy and security of confidential medical data of the participants. Widely implementing blockchain-derived PHRs enables pharmaceutical companies to search the global populations to rapidly spot the proper sample of varied participants worldwide. Ultimately, blockchain techniques could secure patient data, significantly grow exchanging data worldwide, and highly minimize clinical trials' load, complexity, and expenses [30].

4.4.3 Fighting Fake Medications

The pharmaceutical industry devotes enormous sums of money and proceeds in an exhausting process to manufacture and market drug products. However, the counterfeit drug market is growing each year worldwide and is valued in billions of dollars.

In rising markets, 10–30% of prescription drugs are usually fake, ranging from wrong constituents to wrong quantities of constituents. Antibiotics are among the most frequently counterfeit drugs that are purchased online [32].

Missing transparency in the supply chain and authenticity in drug products is the origin of pharmaceutical fraud worldwide where the lack of transparency makes it challenging to identify the root of the fraud, validate product authenticity or determine the poor players who committed the offenses. Therefore, the complete operation, from manufacturing to quality assurance to distribution, needs to be safeguarded in an unbreakable dataset with every entry cryptographically signed and coded. Blockchain techniques supply such potential and subsequent transparency. Hence, pharmaceutical companies are obviously committed to fighting fake drugs besides saving lives threatened by side effects and adverse reactions. In 2017, stakeholders of reputable pharmaceutical companies started the MediLedge blockchain project that facilitates track and trace functionality to members of the pharmaceutical supply chain. Preliminary pilots are promising and show that a blockchain-driven intervention would allow compliance with the Drug Supply Chain Security Act (DSCSA) meanwhile enhancing processes and minimizing the supply of fake drugs [19, 27].

4.4.4 Enhancing 3-D Printing of Medications

The US Food and Drug Administration (FDA) has issued directions in 2017 about using 3-D printing for personalized medications that may be printed by non-conventional producers such as in a healthcare facility. The data of patients should be managed properly before the 3-D medication printing could turn into an effective approach to produce personalized medications per request [33]. Delivering personalized medications is associated with the volume and quality of accessible clinical information on patients. Data on a patient, particularly omics (like epigenomics, genomics, metabolomics, and proteomics), the microbiome, and allergy profile, are vital to finding the accurate kinds and doses of medicines for a certain set of symptoms. Prospective public health data is critical as well to learn about the likely results from various medicines taking into account the patient's age, sex, race, among other variables. Though, now accessing such special kinds of data for a certain patient is challenging since data is disparate among multiple health caregivers. Central frameworks have not yet been reliable since data housed with several patient records is an obstacle and a playground for intruders.

A blockchain-derived PHR encoded with the biometrics of an individual may offer security via a changeless blockchain ledger for logging transactions that would reduce manipulating data. Likewise, blockchain techniques could facilitate exchanging prospective data, producing valuable databases between multiple population reservoirs. Hence, it could be practical to apply Machine Learning (ML) and Artificial Intelligence (AI) techniques on the data to identify quickly the optimum kinds of medications and the doses of active constituents tailored as required per patient. Combining outcomes from ML and AI with a 3-D medication printer enables printing a patient's personalized medication at a physician clinic, a hospital, or a pharmacy [30].

4.4.5 Cryptopharmaceuticals

Applying information-rich models enables sterilizing every dosage unit, check-in after production, and check-out of the product while the patient is administering the prescribed dosage unit. Such models will allow scanning the product by a smartphone to link the products to the IoT and to the health system, whereas AI is adding to the management and doses adjustments decisions [3, 34]. Such digital products are specific and customized for every patient enabling applying the blockchain-based health system [35] (Figure 4.1).

Cryptopharmaceuticals is a blockchain principle for pharmaceutical dosage units where every recent ledger includes the distinctive information for a certain product, revealed as a hash by the producer in the check-in and by the patient in the check-out; hence, every ledger includes a cryptographic hash of the preceding ledger cascading all the ledgers in a non-modifiable mode [35, 36]. Nørfeldt proposed incorporating pharmaceutical products into an IoT-based health system allowing a technological framework for merging ML-driven diagnosis with the patient's data, involving point-of-care sensor data and health records and, eventually producing a safe chain of serialized individualized products. Programming platforms have been used to create an open-source code along with the freely available Android and Apple MedBlockChain application where it has been engineered so that every screen shows four distinct user views: manufacture, patient monitoring, and blockchain allowing accessing information in every workflow level according to whether the user is a healthcare provider, patient, health system, or producer of the medicinal product. However, the latest data on the influences of data breaches suggests that cybersecurity would be among the highly significant challenges to the future health system [37].

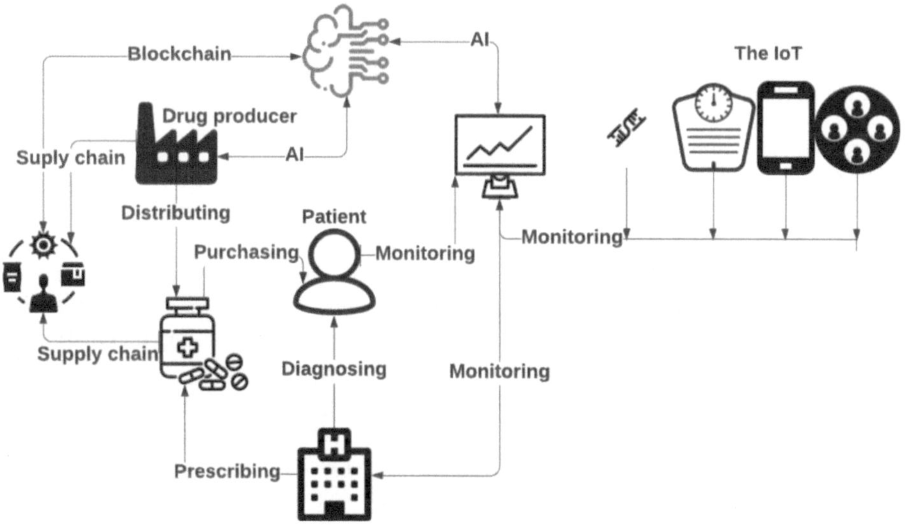

FIGURE 4.1 The future of managing patients via producing personalized medications per need incorporating blockchain for all produced and purchased pharmaceutical products into a central healthcare system.

4.5 DISCUSSIONS

According to the Office for Science suggestions, patients' records can be operated via a decentralized blockchain rather than be safeguarded in a central database. Blockchain decreases the risk of unauthorized access through protocols governing the methods and the people or entities allowed to access such data. For example, a secretary of a primary care facility might only access limited essential information about a patient, such as their name and address. A doctor would have complete access to all medical information [14, 27]. Patients could access their own records as well and even interact with them in a moderated manner. Suggestions include allowing patients to specify preferences of treatment or a list of family members who could participate in decisions concerning their own health. Consent can be moderated and documented easily in this manner. This applies to people keeping track of their records regularly and also to people with a complicated medical history who need to decide on emergency conditions [38].

The communication between the public and private healthcare facilities would be easier. So far these facilities use their own documenting systems. Access to each other is complicated and most times requires arduous bureaucratic procedures and hand transfer of data. Providing patients with the option to allow access to their records contained on a blockchain system to all legal healthcare providers, including private healthcare entities, has been regarded as a significant asset [16]. This has already been implemented in Estonia, where a data security start-up, Guardtime, was established. This collaboration deploys a blockchain-based system safeguarding over one million individual healthcare records. With Guardtime's keyless signature infrastructure blockchain integrated into the Estonian eHealth Foundation's database, patients and practitioners will have real-time access to the records. Similarly, IBM Watson Health announced in 2017 a collaboration with the US FDA in defining a secure, efficient, and scalable exchange of health data via blockchain modalities [27].

4.6 LIMITATIONS

George Bernard Shaw has stated that, "the single biggest problem with communication is the illusion that it is happening". Similarly, the single biggest problem with blockchain modalities can be the fact that people who are not trained and familiarized with this technology expect and are expected to implement it in their working conditions achieving formidable results rapidly [39]. Blockchain literacy is an important obstacle. Not only practitioners and patients but also decision-makers ought to be aware of its properties and limitations. Few governments have released policies regarding the implementation of blockchain, let alone that the legal implications of cryptocurrency in countries such as the United States (US), Russia, and France have probably cultivated some mistrust [40]. In terms of policymaking, the involvement of international institutions or political schemes such as the United Nations (UN), the World Health Organization (WHO), or the European Union (EU) can increase interest in blockchain among national governments and healthcare systems. Policymaking carries inherent obstacles as well though. Blockchain addresses the need for security and confidentiality [41, 42].

Apart from political institutions, academic institutions may also be associated with obstacles. Blockchain has a strong industrial or start-up profile, while in many countries the collaboration between academia and industry is heavily disregarded. In the same frame, usually universities come up with concepts and technology that need industrial support to grow. Introducing the blockchain concept in academia and educating educators there to pass the word to their students is quite a challenge given the busy schedule and insecurity of faculty members to switch from their regular teaching and research field to something new [38].

4.7 CONCLUSIONS

The future of managing patients requires producing personalized medications per need incorporating the IoT with blockchain for all produced and purchased pharmaceutical products into a central healthcare system. Blockchain techniques have a promising impact on investigating a lifelong medication history, minimizing drug counterfeiting, and promoting affordable virtual clinical trials leading to an innovative era of individualized medicine. Cryptopharmaceuticals enables information-rich models of pharmaceuticals to be linked in a patient-specific blockchain for individual dosage units where it is applied for integrating such novel pharmaceutical products into an IoT-based health system. The resulting strong blockchain of individual medication history will facilitate preventing counterfeit products and allow advanced logistic interventions in the drug industry along with raising patient engagement. However, despite the additional values that blockchain brings such as safeguarding integrity and confidentiality and subsequently producing reliable data, there are still concerns regarding the vulnerabilities of blockchain and the inadequate digital literacy of the users, along with incentives, attacks, and key management issues. Cybersecurity would be among the highly significant challenges to the future health system.

REFERENCES

[1] Letai A. Functional Precision Cancer Medicine—Moving beyond Pure Genomics. *Nat Med* 2017;23:1028–35. https://doi.org/10.1038/nm.4389.

[2] Li Q, Zhang L-N, Tao X-M, Ding X. Review of Flexible Temperature Sensing Networks for Wearable Physiological Monitoring. *Adv Healthc Mater* 2017;6:1601371. https://doi.org/10.1002/adhm.201601371.

[3] Dimitrov DV. Medical Internet of Things and Big Data in Healthcare. *Healthc Inform Res* 2016;22:156–63. https://doi.org/10.4258/hir.2016.22.3.156.

[4] Bouton CE, Shaikhouni A, Annetta NV, Bockbrader MA, Friedenberg DA, Nielson DM, et al. Restoring Cortical Control of Functional Movement in a Human with Quadriplegia. *Nature* 2016;533:247–50. https://doi.org/10.1038/nature17435.

[5] Shinbane JS, Saxon LA. Digital Monitoring and Care: Virtual Medicine. *Trends Cardiovasc Med* 2016;26:722–30. https://doi.org/10.1016/j.tcm.2016.05.007.

[6] Chen JH, Asch SM. Machine Learning and Prediction in Medicine — Beyond the Peak of Inflated Expectations. *N Engl J Med* 2017;376:2507–9. https://doi.org/10.1056/NEJMp1702071.

[7] Komorowski M, Celi LA, Badawi O, Gordon AC, Faisal AA. The Artificial Intelligence Clinician Learns Optimal Treatment Strategies for Sepsis in Intensive Care. *Nat Med* 2018;24:1716–20. https://doi.org/10.1038/s41591-018-0213-5.

[8] Obermeyer Z, Emanuel EJ. Predicting the Future — Big Data, Machine Learning, and Clinical Medicine. *N Engl J Med* 2016;375:1216–9. https://doi.org/10.1056/NEJMp1606181.

[9] Rantanen J, Khinast J. The Future of Pharmaceutical Manufacturing Sciences. *J Pharm Sci* 2015;104:3612–38. https://doi.org/10.1002/jps.24594.

[10] Allison G, Cain YT, Cooney C, Garcia T, Bizjak TG, Holte O, et al. Regulatory and Quality Considerations for Continuous Manufacturing May 20–21, 2014 Continuous Manufacturing Symposium. *J Pharm Sci* 2015;104:803–12. https://doi.org/10.1002/jps.24324.

[11] Nasr MM, Krumme M, Matsuda Y, Trout BL, Badman C, Mascia S, et al. Regulatory Perspectives on Continuous Pharmaceutical Manufacturing: Moving From Theory to Practice: September 26-27, 2016, International Symposium on the Continuous Manufacturing of Pharmaceuticals. *J Pharm Sci* 2017;106:3199–206. https://doi.org/10.1016/j.xphs.2017.06.015.

[12] Edinger M, Bar-Shalom D, Sandler N, Rantanen J, Genina N. QR Encoded Smart Oral Dosage Forms by Inkjet Printing. *Int J Pharm* 2018;536:138–45. https://doi.org/10.1016/j.ijpharm.2017.11.052.

[13] Rajan D, Visser M. Quantum Blockchain Using Entanglement in Time. *Quantum Rep* 2019;1:3–11. https://doi.org/10.3390/quantum1010002.

[14] Zubaydi HD, Chong Y-W, Ko K, Hanshi SM, Karuppayah S. A Review on the Role of Blockchain Technology in the Healthcare Domain. *Electronics* 2019;8:679. https://doi.org/10.3390/electronics8060679.

[15] HPECio. Blockchain Technology. Hpeclo 2019. https://hpec.io/how-it-works/ (accessed May 3, 2020).

[16] Yue X, Wang H, Jin D, Li M, Jiang W. Healthcare Data Gateways: Found Healthcare Intelligence on Blockchain with Novel Privacy Risk Control. *J Med Syst* 2016;40:218. https://doi.org/10.1007/s10916-016-0574-6.

[17] Irving G, Holden J. How Blockchain-Timestamped Protocols Could Improve the Trustworthiness of Medical Science. *F1000Research* 2017;5. https://doi.org/10.12688/f1000research.8114.3.

[18] Nugent T, Upton D, Cimpoesu M. Improving Data Transparency in Clinical Trials using Blockchain Smart Contracts. *F1000Research* 2016;5:2541. https://doi.org/10.12688/f1000research.9756.1.

[19] Kim S, Park H, Lee J. Word2vec-based Latent Semantic Analysis (W2V-LSA) for Topic Modeling: A Study on Blockchain Technology Trend Analysis. *Expert Syst Appl* 2020;152:113401. https://doi.org/10.1016/j.eswa.2020.113401.

[20] Tariq N, Asim M, Al-Obeidat F, Zubair Farooqi M, Baker T, Hammoudeh M, et al. The Security of Big Data in Fog-Enabled IoT Applications Including Blockchain: A Survey. *Sensors* 2019;19:1788. https://doi.org/10.3390/s19081788.

[21] Islam SMR, Kwak D, Kabir MDH, Hossain M, Kwak K-S. The Internet of Things for Health Care: A Comprehensive Survey. *IEEE Access* 2015;3:678–708. https://doi.org/10.1109/ACCESS.2015.2437951.

[22] Sharma M, Singh G, Singh R. An Advanced Conceptual Diagnostic Healthcare Framework for Diabetes and Cardiovascular Disorders. *ICST Trans Scalable Inf Syst* 2018;5:154828. https://doi.org/10.4108/eai.19-6-2018.154828.

[23] Shukla S, Hassan MF, Khan MK, Jung LT, Awang A. An Analytical Model to Minimize the Latency in Healthcare Internet-of-Things in Fog Computing Environment. *PLOS ONE* 2019;14:e0224934. https://doi.org/10.1371/journal.pone.0224934.

[24] Gopal G, Suter-Crazzolara C, Toldo L, Eberhardt W. Digital Transformation in Healthcare - Architectures of Present and Future Information Technologies. *Clin Chem Lab Med* 2019;57:328–35. https://doi.org/10.1515/cclm-2018-0658.

[25] Islam N, Faheem Y, Din IU, Talha M, Guizani M, Khalil M. A Blockchain-based Fog Computing Framework for Activity Recognition as an Application to e-Healthcare Services. *Future Gener Comput Syst* 2019;100:569–78. https://doi.org/10.1016/j.future.2019.05.059.

[26] Jagadeeswari V, Subramaniyaswamy V, Logesh R, Vijayakumar V. A Study on Medical Internet of Things and Big Data in Personalized Healthcare System. *Health Inf Sci Syst* 2018;6:14. https://doi.org/10.1007/s13755-018-0049-x.
[27] Birch V, White L, Critchley P. Blockchain Technology: Application in Life Sciences and Healthcare Sectors. 2019. https://www.nortonrosefulbright.com/en/knowledge/publications/cb048fa5/blockchain-technology-application-in-life-sciences-and-healthcare-sectors (accessed June 2, 2020).
[28] Fearn N. IoT Smart Fridge Revolutionising Vaccine Care. Internet Bus 2016. https://internetofbusiness.com/iot-smart-fridge-vaccine-care/ (accessed June 2, 2020).
[29] Özdemir V, Hekim N. Birth of Industry 5.0: Making Sense of Big Data with Artificial Intelligence, "The Internet of Things" and Next-Generation Technology Policy. *OMICS J Integr Biol* 2018;22:65–76. https://doi.org/10.1089/omi.2017.0194.
[30] Woods J, Iyengar-Emens R. Blockchain to Secure a More Personalized Pharma. GEN - Genet Eng Biotechnol News. 2019. https://www.genengnews.com/insights/blockchain-to-secure-a-more-personalized-pharma/ (accessed March 10, 2020).
[31] Mantel-Undark B. The Search for New Drugs is Coming to your House. Fast Co 2018. https://www.fastcompany.com/90229910/virtual-clinical-trials-are-bringing-drug-development-home (accessed May 25, 2020).
[32] Health Research Funding. 20 Shocking Counterfeit Drugs Statistics. HRF 2014. https://healthresearchfunding.org/20-shocking-counterfeit-drugs-statistics/ (accessed March 9, 2020).
[33] U.S. Food & Drug Administration. Statement by FDA Commissioner Scott Gottlieb, M.D., on FDA ushering in new era of 3D printing of medical products; provides guidance to manufacturers of medical devices. 2020. https://www.fda.gov/news-events/press-announcements/statement-fda-commissioner-scott-gottlieb-md-fda-ushering-new-era-3d-printing-medical-products (accessed May 26, 2020).
[34] Miotto R, Wang F, Wang S, Jiang X, Dudley JT. Deep Learning for Healthcare: Review, Opportunities and Challenges. *Brief Bioinform* 2018;19:1236–46. https://doi.org/10.1093/bib/bbx044.
[35] Zhang M, Ji Y. Blockchain for Healthcare Records: A Data Perspective. *PeerJ Inc.*; 2018. 1-5 https://doi.org/10.7287/peerj.preprints.26942v1.
[36] Preneel B. Cryptographic Hash Functions: Theory and Practice. In: Soriano M, Qing S, López J, editors. *Inf Commun Secur*, Berlin, Heidelberg: Springer; 2010, p. 1–3. https://doi.org/10.1007/978-3-642-17650-0_1.
[37] Nørfeldt L, Bøtker J, Edinger M, Genina N, Rantanen J. Cryptopharmaceuticals: Increasing the Safety of Medication by a Blockchain of Pharmaceutical Products. *J Pharm Sci* 2019;108:2838–41. https://doi.org/10.1016/j.xphs.2019.04.025.
[38] McGhin T, Choo K-KR, Liu CZ, He D. Blockchain in Healthcare Applications: Research Challenges and Opportunities. *J Netw Comput Appl* 2019;135:62–75. https://doi.org/10.1016/j.jnca.2019.02.027.
[39] Cirillo F, Wu F-J, Solmaz G, Kovacs E. Embracing the Future Internet of Things. *Sensors* 2019;19. https://doi.org/10.3390/s19020351.
[40] Cao S, Zhang G, Liu P, Zhang X, Neri F. Cloud-Assisted Secure eHealth Systems for Tamper-proofing EHR via Blockchain. *Inf Sci* 2019;485:427–40. https://doi.org/10.1016/j.ins.2019.02.038.
[41] Baldini G, Botterman M, Neisse R, Tallacchini M. Ethical Design in the Internet of Things. *Sci Eng Ethics* 2018;24:905–25. https://doi.org/10.1007/s11948-016-9754-5.
[42] Boyd D, Crawford K. Critical Questions for Big Data. *Inf Commun Soc* 2012;15:662–79. https://doi.org/10.1080/1369118X.2012.678878.

5 Wearable/Implantable Devices for Monitoring Systems

Pawan Kumar[1] *and Shabana Urooj*[2]
[1,2]Department of Electrical Engineering, School of Engineering, Gautam Buddha University, Greater Noida–201310, India

CONTENTS

5.1 Introduction ... 64
5.2 Biomedical Telemetry ... 64
5.2.1 Implantable/Sensing Antennas ... 64
5.2.2 Electronics Circuitry ... 65
5.2.3 Biosensors and Bio-actuators ... 65
5.2.4 Insulations ... 65
5.2.5 Characterization and Experiments ... 66
5.2.6 Human Body ... 66
5.2.7 Channel Propagation ... 66
5.2.8 Base Station ... 66
5.3 Application of Antennas in the Medical Field ... 66
5.3.1 Diagnostics ... 66
5.3.1.1 Magnetic Resonance Imaging ... 66
5.3.1.2 Wireless Capsule Endoscopy ... 67
5.3.2 Therapy ... 67
5.3.2.1 Cancer Treatment Using Hyperthermia ... 67
5.3.2.2 Coagulation Therapy ... 67
5.4 Use of Antennas for Diagnosis ... 68
5.4.1 Implantable Antennas ... 69
5.4.1.1 Design Procedure of Implantable Antennas ... 70
5.4.2 Ingestible Antennas ... 72
5.4.2.1 Design Requirements of Ingestible Antennas ... 73
5.4.2.2 Design Methodology of Ingestible Antennas ... 73
5.4.3 Wearable Antennas ... 74
5.4.3.1 Ordinary Wearable Designs ... 75
5.4.3.2 Textile Antenna Designs ... 76
5.4.3.3 Designing Wearable Antennas ... 77
5.4.3.4 Analysis of Wearable Antennas ... 77

5.5 Application of Antennas for Disease Treatment 78
5.5.1 Hyperthermia Therapy 78
5.5.2 Coagulation Therapy 79
5.6 Future Trends 79
5.7 Conclusion 79
References 79

5.1 INTRODUCTION

Microwaves are electromagnetic radiations with frequency ranging from 300 MHz and 300 GHz. Due to their basic properties like penetration, absorption, reflection, high-frequency and short wavelength, they find applications in disease diagnosis (imaging process), therapy (treatment of cancer using hyperthermia) and prevention [1, 2]. Wireless transmission of signals over a distance allows patient health to be monitored remotely. This eliminates the need to keep the patient in the hospital for many days, which in turn reduces the total cost incurred by the patient. This concept is already being used in glucose monitoring, endoscopy, insulin pumps and for testing various other body fluids.

Keeping this in view, the rise in the research on antennas and the signal propagation for body communication systems, an IEEE 802.15 standardization group was set up for standardizing applications focusing on off-, in- and on-body communication. The in-body equipment are used to communicate between the medical devices implanted in the body (for example, WCE) and the on-body nodes. Off-body communication is the link connecting body-worn devices and the receiver unit in the surrounding area [3]. Body-Centric Communication (BCC) occupies an important place in Body Area Networks (BANs) and Personal Area Networks (PANs).

5.2 BIOMEDICAL TELEMETRY

The use of implantable devices such as pacemakers, antennas, swallowable pills for monitoring different internal parameters of the body is increasing day-by-day. Such devices usually consist of an antenna system and power supply unit [4], so that after recording the signals, the information can be transmitted to the receiver unit present outside the human body.

Figure 5.1 illustrates an example of human healthcare monitoring system. The healthcare monitoring system consists of the following components: implantable/sensing antennas, electronics circuitry, biosensors and bio-actuators, insulations, characterization and experiments, human body, channel propagation, and base station.

5.2.1 Implantable/Sensing Antennas

Antennas are the main component of the implantable devices, as they help in the bidirectional communication (communication between implantable device and external receiver unit). Different types of antenna designs have been studied by the researchers, but the patch antennas are popularly used for implantable

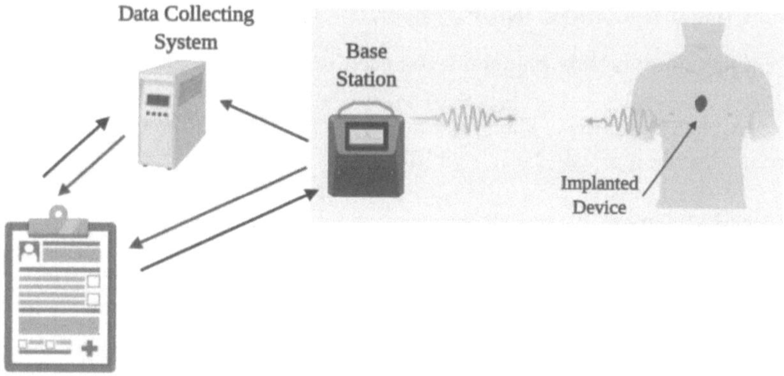

FIGURE 5.1 Schematic of a healthcare monitoring system.

applications as they are low-profile, flexible and conformal [5–7]. These properties of the patch antenna lead to compactness and their easy integration into the implantable systems, as they can be molded according to the profile of the implantable appliance.

5.2.2 Electronics Circuitry

The electrical/electronic components of a wireless implant system permit the operation and provide the signal processing and data transmission among the base station and the implanted device. The battery or the power supplying unit defines the lifetime of the implanted device. Research has been done on various approaches to increase the life span of the implantable system such as internal power supplies, harvesting of energy, wireless power transfer, etc. [8, 9].

5.2.3 Biosensors and Bio-actuators

The biosensors and bio-actuators contained in the implantable system may vary depending on the application for which the implantable device is being designed. This also helps in deciding the position of the implant inside the human body. Various monitoring sensors for monitoring different physiological parameters such as pH, temperature, glucose, etc., or the active systems (which monitor some parameter and perform some action based on their reading things like drug delivery apparatus) are being investigated and used.

5.2.4 Insulations

The wireless implantable device should be properly insulated in a biocompatible material to prevent any adverse reaction and rejection of the implant by the body. The implant should be prevented from coming in direct contact with body fluids, which are conductive in nature; otherwise the device may short-circuit.

5.2.5 Characterization and Experiments

Every component which is planned to be used in the healthcare monitoring system should be characterized to validate its performance and to make sure that it conforms to all the regulations. The system is tested in vitro and then on animal models (in vivo testing) before using it in real life [10].

5.2.6 Human Body

The implantable device is fixed in the human body to monitor various physiological parameters. The implantable device should be designed keeping in mind the complex, highly lossy nature of the human body and conductive nature of biofluids. Proper characterization of the device properties should be performed in human tissue-mimicking models before its actual application in a real-time environment.

5.2.7 Channel Propagation

Channel propagation handles the propagation of signals from the wireless implanted system to the receiving terminals. The receiving system processes the received data and extracts useful information from it.

5.2.8 Base Station

The base station consists of numerous sub-systems:

a. A control module to drive and control the functioning of the complete system.
b. A receiver module containing antennas to receive the signal from the implanted system.
c. An internet modulator/demodulator or apparatus to collect and transfer the information from the data collecting system.

5.3 APPLICATION OF ANTENNAS IN THE MEDICAL FIELD

Primarily, the antennas are used in medicine for two purposes [11]: diagnostics and therapy.

5.3.1 Diagnostics

In diagnostics, the electromagnetic energy is transmitted and received by the antennas to measure various physiological parameters in the human body.

5.3.1.1 Magnetic Resonance Imaging

The antenna is a key component of various medical instruments, which are used for diagnosis such as Magnetic Resonance Imaging (MRI). The electromagnetic field formed by the antennas of the MRI machine is focused on the part of the human body to be diagnosed. The spin of the hydrogen nuclei of the water molecules present in the body part to be diagnosed is aligned on the application of a strong field by the MRI machine. Upon discontinuing the field on the body part, the hydrogen nuclei will

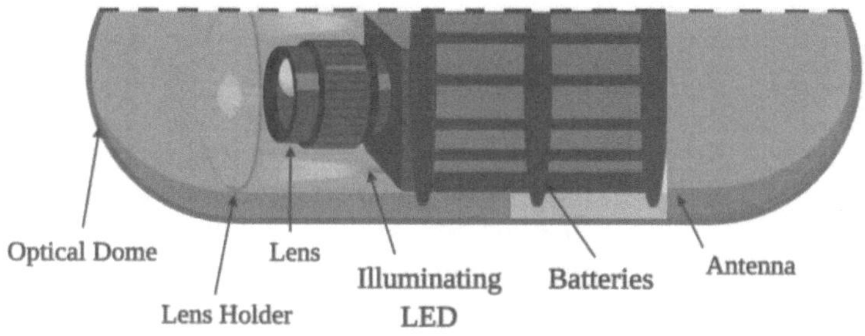

FIGURE 5.2 Capsule endoscopy pill.

return to their original spin and release the energy gained in this process. The gained energy emitted in the form of a nuclear magnetic resonance signal is measured by the receiver antennas and converted into an image for further analysis by the doctor.

5.3.1.2 Wireless Capsule Endoscopy

As the name suggests, the Wireless Capsule Endoscopy (WCE) demonstrates the picture of whole gastrointestinal (GI) tract without any cable. This technique is useful and finds its application in the detection of various gastrointestinal diseases like GI tumors, cancers, Obscure Gastrointestinal Bleeding (OGIB), Celiac disease, Crohn's disease [12]. The layout of a capsule endoscopy pill is represented in Figure 5.2. WCE is a miniaturized pill with a camera, battery, light source and a transmitter, which transmits signals to the receiver. The patient swallows the miniaturized capsule, which then captures and sends images as it moves through the GI tract due to the natural movement of the tract. After moving through the whole GI tract, the capsule will automatically come out of the patient's body and can be used to retrieve and interpret the information.

5.3.2 Therapy

5.3.2.1 Cancer Treatment Using Hyperthermia

This process involves the heating of tumors, which damages the membrane of the tumor cells and results in the death of the cells. The schematic of local hyperthermia system is illustrated Figure 5.3. Firstly, the site of the tumor cells should be located specifically. Once the position of cancerous tissue is known, then the antenna is used to focus electromagnetic waves on the cancerous tissue and generate heat. The antenna emits microwaves, which enter the cancerous cells and make the water molecules of the cells vibrate with high speed. Due to the vibration in water molecules, heat is generated owing to the friction between different water molecules, which kills the cancerous cells. This treatment can be used along with chemotherapy or X-ray irradiation. The block diagram in Figure 5.4 shows the details of hyperthermia therapy.

5.3.2.2 Coagulation Therapy

In this approach, the antenna is positioned at the center of the cancerous tissue and by using the heat produced from microwave radiations, the cancerous tissues are destroyed. In this process, when the temperature crosses 60°C, coagulation happens

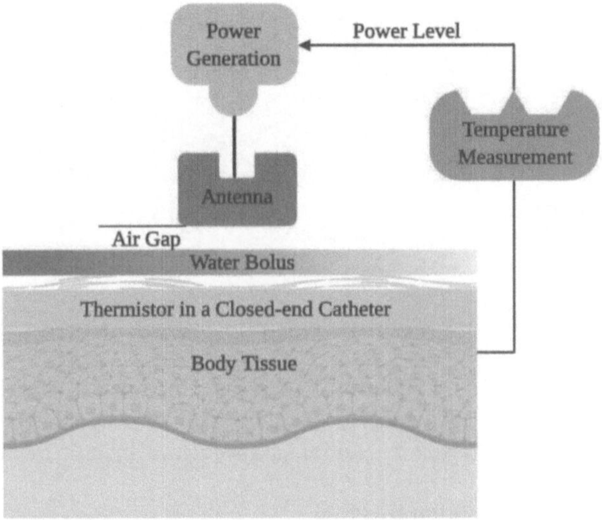

FIGURE 5.3 Schematic of local hyperthermia system.

in the exposed region including cancer cells, which results in the death of cancer cells. The various types of antennas used for microwave heating are presented in Figure 5.5.

5.4 USE OF ANTENNAS FOR DIAGNOSIS

Nowadays, antennas are playing a key role in the diagnosis process. The different types of antennas being used for diagnosis of different diseases are shown in Figure 5.6.

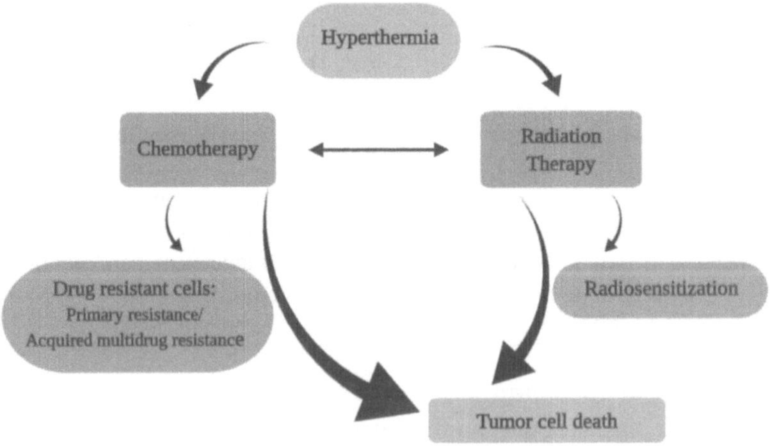

FIGURE 5.4 Block diagram representing hyperthermia therapy.

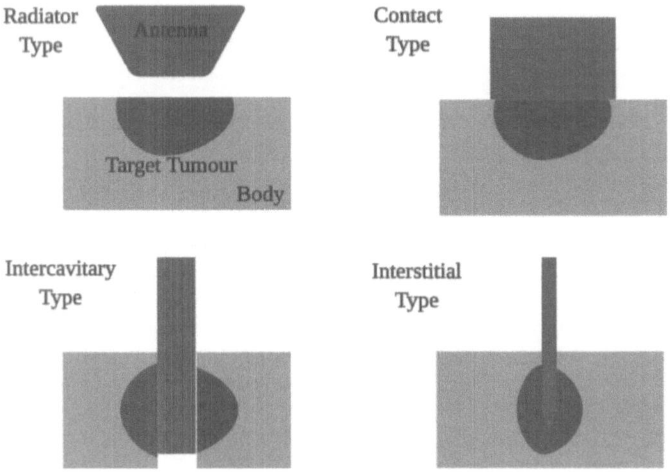

FIGURE 5.5 Various types of antennas used for microwave heating.

5.4.1 Implantable Antennas

These antennas are implanted inside the body for constant monitoring of different body parameters such as blood glucose level, brain activity, cardiac activity, etc. [13, 14]. These antennas must be designed by using some biocompatible material or should be enclosed in some biocompatible material to avoid any adverse reaction and its rejection by the body. If the metallization of the implantable antenna comes in direct contact with the human body fluids, which are conductive in nature,

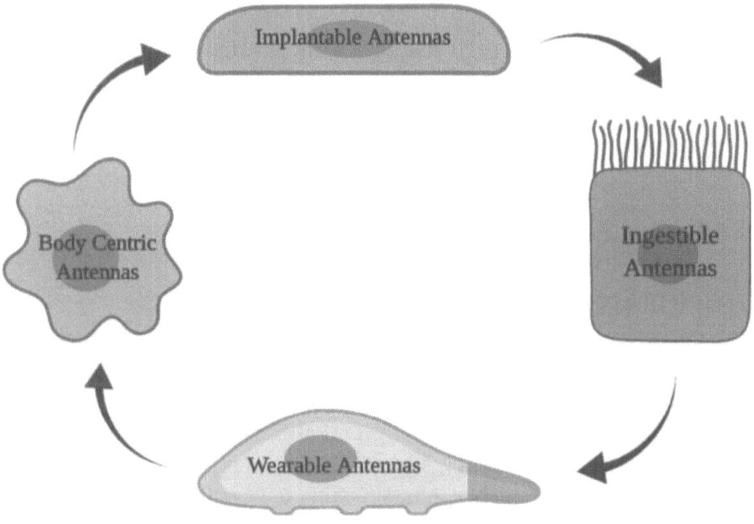

FIGURE 5.6 Different types of antennas used for diagnosis.

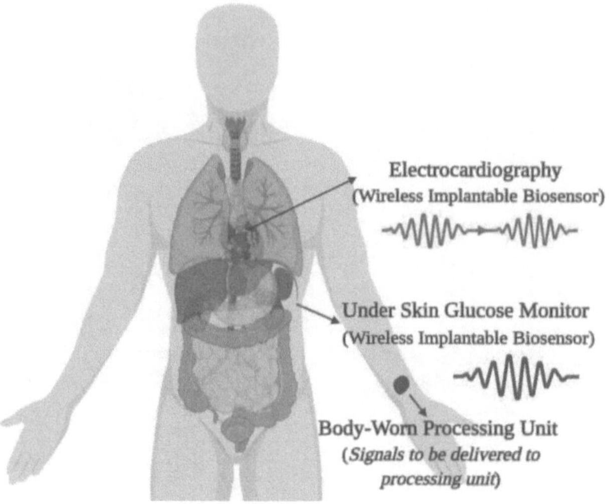

FIGURE 5.7 Uses of implantable antennas.

then short-circuit may happen. To avoid any such incident, the antenna set-up can be covered with superstrate material/layer of Macor, alumina ceramic, polytetrafluoroethylene (PTFE), etc. These materials act as a separating layer between the human tissues and the radiator in addition to providing the biocompatibility property. Figure 5.7 shows different uses of implantable antennas.

The various design requirements of implantable antennas are:

a. Characterization of the implanted antenna should be done.
b. The antenna should be low profile, which matches with the environment of the body.
c. Evaluation of radiation performance of the compact, low-profile antenna should be done by studies like radiation efficiency and return loss.
d. The performance of the transmission link between the implanted antenna and the recipient unit should be assessed using various techniques.

Table 5.1 gives the details of various implantable antennas being used by the researchers in the last few years.

5.4.1.1 Design Procedure of Implantable Antennas

Firstly, the numerical simulation tool (Ansys HFSS, CST Microwave Studio, IE3D, etc.) is used to simulate the structure and evaluate characteristics of the antenna, which works in Medical Implant Communication System (MICS) (0.402–0.405 GHz) and Industrial, Scientific and Medical (ISM) (2.4–2.48 GHz) bands. After optimizing the antenna parameters through simulation tool, fabrication of antenna is done and the behavior of the antenna is evaluated using gels as they can mimic the electrical characteristics of human body tissues. The design procedure of the implantable antenna is explained in Figure 5.8.

TABLE 5.1
Various Types of Implantable Antennas Reported in the Literature

Ref.	Resonating Band (GHz)	Substrate Layout/Radiator Shape	Implantation	Substrate	Volume (mm³)
[15]	0.402–0.405	Rectangular/ Spiral	Skin	Rogers 3210	6144
[16]	0.402–0.405, 2.4–2.48	Square/SRR coupled	Skin	ARLON 1000	1375.4
[17]	0.402–0.405	Square/Spiral	Vitreous humor	Rogers 3210	273.6
[18]	0.402–0.405	Circular/Slotted	Skin	Rogers 3210	149.2
[19]	0.402–0.405	Rectangular/ Meandered	Skin	Rogers 3210	1200
[20]	0.402–0.405	Rectangular/ Waffle	Muscle	RT/Duroid 6002	6480
[21]	0.402–0.405	Circular/ Meandered	Skin	Rogers 3210	110.4
[22]	0.402–0.405	Square/Spiral	Skin	Rogers 3210	190
[23]	0.402–0.405	Circular/Slotted	Skin	Rogers 3210	335.8
[24]	0.402–0.405	Circular/ Meandered	Skin	Alumina	32.7

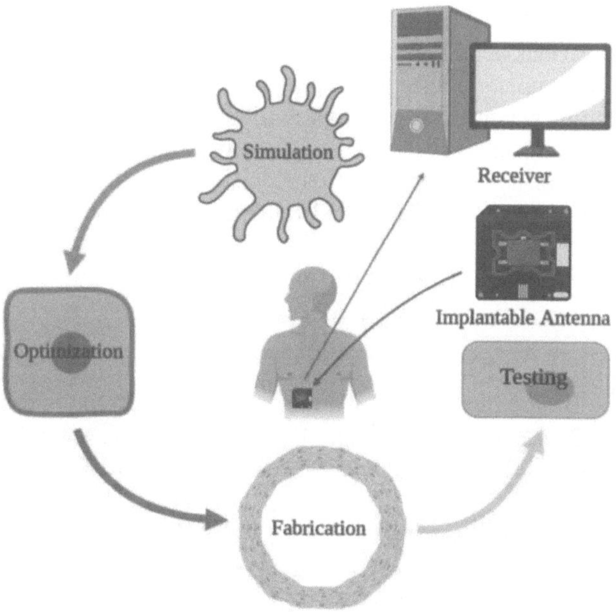

FIGURE 5.8 Design procedure of the implantable antennas.

Characterization must be performed for the tissue-mimicking material using different techniques. The Specific Absorption Rate (SAR) studies should be performed before proceeding with the in vitro testing of the system. Besides tissues, the radiation of the implantable antenna should pass through the skin to reach the collector present outside the human body so the characterization of the material (a mix of Triton X-114, diethylene glycol butyl ether, salt and deionized water can be used as skin mimicking material), which possess the same properties as human skin can be performed. After materials characterization, studies in animal models such as rats must be performed.

Recently, various researchers have proposed different implantable antenna designs for MICS/ISM band applications [25–30]. In [25], a low-profile Coplanar Waveguide (CPW)-fed V-shaped implantable antenna etched on FR-4 substrate was proposed. This antenna was reported for ISM band biomedical applications and can be positioned on various human tissues such as skin, fat and muscles. IE3D software was used to simulate the antenna design. In [26], a dual-band antenna for implantable neuro-microsystem was reported. The operating frequencies of the antenna were 433.9 and 542.4 MHz. The SAR study of the antenna was performed by the authors using the solution which mimics the properties of the tissues. In [27], the authors proposed a dipole, patch and inverted-F antennas to help paralyzed patients. The device was designed in such a way that it can be placed in the buccal space of the mouth to issue commands using the user-decided gestures of the tongue. This implantable antenna has a compact design enclosed in an arc-shaped device, better bandwidth and gain in comparison to other implantable antennas reported in the past. In [28], planar inverted-F and dipole antennas working at ISM band were reported. These antennas were part of the device placed in the mouth of paralyzed patients, which identifies the signals generated by the voluntary movement of the tongue. The received signals were processed and various activities like the movement of the wheelchair, operation of mobile phone or computer device have been carried out. In [29], a compact CPW-fed dual spiral alumina antenna was proposed for implantable applications. The antenna operates in ISM band and was tested using human models. It possesses higher gain, low return loss with good impedance matching. In [30], the authors presented the design of an ultra-compact spiral coiled implantable antenna with wireless power transfer capability. The power was transferred from an external transmitter device and an efficiency of 47.2% at a frequency of 39.86 MHz was obtained.

5.4.2 Ingestible Antennas

The antenna is located inside a capsule that moves through the internal organs and digestive tract of the body as illustrated in Figure 5.9. These antennas are useful in diagnosing various GI cancers such as cancer of the oesophagus, liver, small intestine, pancreas, etc.

Techniques are available to track upper (gastroscopy) and lower (colonoscopy) parts of the GI tract, but the middle part of the GI tract which includes the long and highly convoluted small intestine (average 7 meters) is difficult to monitor using these techniques. In such a case, the WCE technique is very helpful to view the whole GI tract. The WCE setup consists of Light-Emitting Diodes (LEDs) for

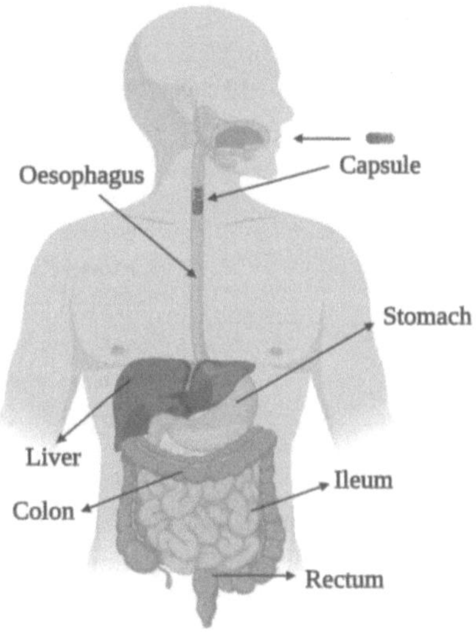

FIGURE 5.9 Ingestible antenna travelling through the digestive tract of the body.

providing light, wireless RF transmitter, antenna, battery and color video camera to capture the internal view of the organs.

The ingestible antennas function in the following frequency bands:

a. MICS (0.402–0.405 GHz)
b. Wireless Medical Telemetry Service (WMTS) (0.608–0.614 GHz, 1.395–1.4 GHz and 1.427–1.432 GHz)
c. ISM (2.4–2.48 GHz)

5.4.2.1 Design Requirements of Ingestible Antennas

In order to perform the design of an ingestible antenna, the following aspect must to be taken into account,

a. The antenna bandwidth should be high so that high-definition images and data of GI tract (for example temperature, oxygen concentration, pH, etc.) can be transmitted.
b. The antenna efficiency should be high to consume less power and transmit data at higher rates.
c. As WCE is fabricated to function inside the human body where body fluids offer a conductive environment, which may affect and change the antenna performance. So, all these factors must be taken into consideration while proposing the antenna design.

5.4.2.2 Design Methodology of Ingestible Antennas

The initial characterization can be performed using the human body model as it mimics the properties of human tissues. The variations of conductivity (0.98 to 1.34 S/m),

TABLE 5.2
Comparison between Probe Endoscopy and Wireless Capsule Endoscopy

Probe Endoscopy	WCE
Poor insertion capability and cannot reach into the middle, highly convoluted small intestine part.	Good insertion capability and can reach/scan the small intestine part.
Unable to reach hidden locations of GI tract.	It can reach hidden locations and provides efficient visualization of complete GI tract.
It cannot diagnose/detect GI tract cancer.	It can diagnose/detect GI tract cancer.
It is painful and can create discomfort.	Not painful/uncomfortable.

dielectric constant (54.81 to 53.55) and frequency (1 to 1.8 GHz) were illustrated in the model shown in [31]. A linearly polarized receiving antenna placed at around 20 cm distance from the model was used for signal detection and characterization. Generally, human body models with single layer are mostly used for simulations due to their simplicity and faster performance, in spite of being less accurate. To evaluate the performance of ingestible antennas, body tissues mimicking fluids (prepared using sugar, salt, cellulose, deionized water, etc.) can be used.

In [31], the authors showed a systematic evaluation and characterization of antenna parameters for two different antenna structures. They used a box model to characterize both antennas individually and showed antenna radiation patterns, polarization, SAR studies and link budget to explain communication of the antenna in the human body with the outside receiver. The researchers in [32] designed magnetic and electric antennas with similar properties and noticed that the magnetic antenna is more efficient than the electric antenna. Also, the magnetic antenna consumes less power which enhances the life of the battery of the endoscopic capsule. In [33], a small spiral-shaped antenna was reported for the endoscopic capsule system and performed experiments in a pig animal model. In addition, a human phantom was used to evaluate and study radiation patterns and resonance characteristics of the proposed system to simulate the high dielectric and lossy environment of the human body. In [34], a conformal small size antenna for MedRadio (0.401–0.406 GHz) band WCE applications was presented. The detailed simulation study was conducted assuming that the capsule was surrounded by human tissues. Table 5.2 provides a comparison between the two popularly used endoscopy techniques (probe and WCE).

5.4.3 Wearable Antennas

Wearable antennas are one of the key research areas of body-centric communications. These types of antennas must have low cost, be lightweight, have simple installation with almost zero maintenance. These types of antennas are useful for people of all age groups and occupations (such as firefighters, military personnel and paramedics) for monitoring purposes. Fabric-based antennas are mainly utilized for wearable applications. In the antenna configuration, the conductive textile elements like Flectron, Zelt and pure copper taffeta fabrics can be employed as the radiator; whereas non-conductive textile elements like fleece, felt and silk can be used as dielectric substrates. The relative permittivity values for these materials are not freely available and need to be measured. The different types of wearable antennas are described below.

5.4.3.1 Ordinary Wearable Designs

Conventional designs such as planar monopoles, dipoles, microstrip patches, Planar Inverted-F Antennas (PIFAs), etc. have been explored and used for the designing of wearable antennas. Due to their low cost and easy fabrication advantages, they are one of the preferred choices for wearable systems. The authors in [35] investigated a PIFA design, which can be positioned on the sleeves and may be used for monitoring purposes. In PIFA, the folded structure is placed parallel to its ground surface. The ground surface acts as a reflector and prevents the antenna radiations from going towards the human body. The same design concept was exploited to design a wearable flexible PIFA (FlexPIFA), which can be placed on the human arm and controlled by a Bluetooth operated system [36]. Figure 5.10 illustrates the possible placement of the PIFA antenna. The following factors are considered while selecting a wearable antenna [37]:

a. Low profile
b. The frequency range must be 100–500 MHz
c. Omni-directional radiation coverage with minimal or no side lobes
d. Vertical or circular polarization
e. Wide return loss bandwidth

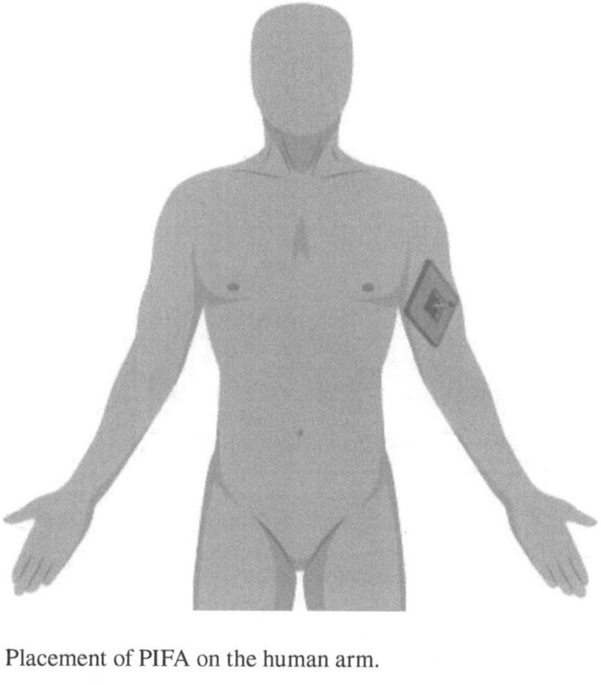

FIGURE 5.10 Placement of PIFA on the human arm.

5.4.3.2 Textile Antenna Designs

The researchers in [38] designed a wearable textile antenna with circular polarization, which accounts for the mobility of the user. In circular polarization, the antenna radiates energy in all the planes from vertical to horizontal direction [39]; so, even if the body coordination changes, the receiver antenna can obtain signals. Polymide spacer fabric (thickness: 6 mm, permittivity: 1.5) was used as the substrate for the antenna design. The radiator and the ground surface were made from the nickel-plated woven textile material. A similar approach was used in [40], where a textile antenna with circular polarization was designed to excite two orthogonally polarized modes in order to improve the signal reception.

One of the most rapidly advancing areas of electromagnetic research is Electromagnetic Band-Gap (EBG). The usage of EBG structure as the ground plane helps in the efficient radiation of the electric current. In [41], the researchers used this concept to design a dual-band wearable structure. The EBG layer on the ground surface improves the radiation behavior of the antenna. Antenna efficiency is high due to the balanced surface current. A textile antenna was designed [42] for providing a short-range wireless communication between the human body and the PAN. The bandwidth was high relative to other classic planar feed antennas [43] due to the use of aperture coupled feeding. Figure 5.11 illustrates the human model with a wearable antenna on woven textile material.

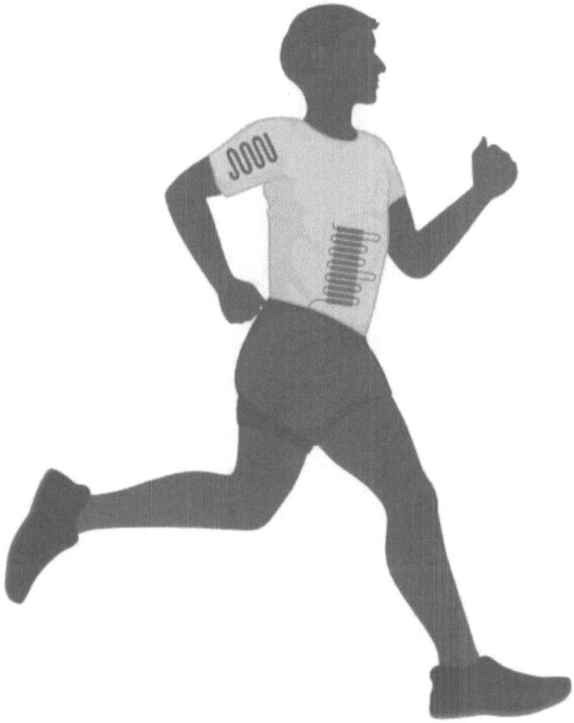

FIGURE 5.11 Wearable antennas on woven textile material.

5.4.3.3 Designing Wearable Antennas

The performance parameters for a wearable antenna depends on the materials and fabrication methods. The material not only influences performance but also radiation properties of the antenna. In fact, textile materials turn out to be better than non-textile ones.

a. Conductive material
   Electro-textile fabrics are created by interpolating threads of ordinary fabric with the threads of conductive metal/polymer. Such fabrics can be used for clothing owing to their flexible, durable and wearable characteristics [44]. In [45], the authors highlighted the importance of conductive fabrics in the fabrication of textile antennas. The conductive fabric should have low resistance (≤1 Ω/square) in order to reduce the losses. Flexibility is also desired in the textile material, for the deformation of the antenna. Aramid woven fabric [46] has also been used as the material for antenna designing due to its flame-resistant property and thus can be integrated into a firefighter's clothes. Metalized nylon fabric with high conductivity was employed as the conductor [47]. It consists of Ni/Cu/Ag layers that provide high conductivity. Additionally, this material is flexible and corrosion-resistant and thus found its application in highly corrosive surroundings.
b. Fabrication method
   The fabrication varies according to the material selected for designing textile antennas and influence the overall cost of the antenna design. In [48], different fabrication methods were reported to design the same microstrip patch antenna. The simplest technique identified after experimentations is to use a copper tape, as it can be easily applied to the dielectric substrates without any additional fabrication step. Conductive spray technique offers more flexibility and can be used for the fabrication of any textile material. The copper tape (conducting element) was used with felt fabric (used as substrate) to construct an E-shaped patch antenna [49].

5.4.3.4 Analysis of Wearable Antennas

Generally, conventional antennas are assessed on parameters like radiation pattern, return loss, efficiency and gain. Usually, the conventional antennas are planar structures due to which no bending characteristic study is needed. But, the study of bending characteristics and other factors is needed to test the performance of the wearable antenna in a body-worn environment. This section will give some details on the measurements that are necessary for examining the performance of the wearable design.

a. Specific absorption rate modeling
   Public concerns and legal requirements about the effects of radiation on human health worldwide make researchers and engineers study the amount of power radiated by the antenna being absorbed by the human body. Two Specific Absorption Rate (SAR) limits are commonly used: IEEE 1.6 W/kg for

any 1 g of tissue [50]; International Commission on Non-Ionizing Radiation Protection (ICNIRP) 2 W/kg for any 10 g of tissue [51]. The SAR modeling was performed using a torso model [52], which was constructed using real MRI and CT image of the human body.

b. Measurement at different bending positions

The performance of the antenna is evaluated by taking measurements at different bending positions. These measurements will help in assessing the behavior of the wearable antenna, especially when the antenna will be used at different places and different bending positions on the body (such as the performance of the antenna when it is worn on the arm). Researchers have already performed S_{11} measurements in different bending positions of the antenna [45]. The antenna was attached around a cylinder and measurements were performed to study the bending characteristics. It was analyzed that the bandwidth decreases and the resonance moves towards lower frequencies in the bending position. This can be overcome by designing an antenna with broad bandwidth so that even if frequency alteration takes place due to bending, then, too, the antenna will function in the desired spectrum range.

c. On-body measurements

Besides the above measurements, where the antenna measurements were taken in the absence of the human body, the on-body measurements need to be performed as well. The position of the antenna on the human body will differ based on its application. Wearable antennas are usually placed on the arm, chest, thigh and back of the human body. The designed antenna in [48] was first placed away from the human body (in free space), then the measurements were carried out on the human arm and chest. From the investigations carried out by various researchers, it is seen that the back of the human body is the most stable position for placing the antenna and taking measurements with least change in orientation as compared to other body parts.

5.5 APPLICATION OF ANTENNAS FOR DISEASE TREATMENT

Nowadays, antennas are not only playing a key role in the diagnosis of various diseases but in the treatment of diseases as well. For example, the antennas can be used in hyperthermia, which adds effectiveness to other therapies like chemotherapy and radiotherapy being given to cancer patients [53]. Antennas can be used in various ways for the treatment of diseases, as shown below.

5.5.1 Hyperthermia Therapy

In hyperthermia, the difference in the sensitivity of normal and tumor cells (to the heat) is exploited. The tumor cells are heated up by increasing temperature to the therapeutic range (42 to 45°C) and protecting the surrounding normal cells from heating at the same time. It is helpful, as it can increase the effectiveness of chemotherapy and radiotherapy given to cancer patients.

5.5.2 Coagulation Therapy

This therapy also involves the heating of targeted cells such as heating of hepatic cells present in the blood clot (for the treatment of hepatocellular carcinoma). Coaxial slot antennas were used for heating tumor cells in the human body. In [54], it was shown that a microwave coaxial slot antenna can be used for hyperthermia therapy of interstitial as well as intracavitary tumor cells. The authors in [53] illustrated the use of antennas in thermal therapies of neck tumors and proved its effectiveness using clinical studies. Previous studies have proved that the coaxial slot antenna can be used to guide the heating effect to burn only the desired cancel cells.

5.6 FUTURE TRENDS

The antenna must have sufficient bandwidth to transmit high-definition images and other diagnosis data like pressure, temperature, oxygen concentration, pH, etc. The antenna must be efficient and must consume less power to extend the lifetime of the battery.

The antennas for WCE should be compact and properly encapsulated in a biocompatible material to prevent any adverse effects during their usage in the human body. Further research is needed to have more control over the movement of the endoscopic capsule, improving the quality and transmission speed of the captured images obtained during the capsule movement. Studies for the development of complex capsule containing therapeutic tools are also required. The development of such a device will help in detecting and treating the diseases of the GI tract (medical robot).

The principle of magnetic induction can be used to transmit power wirelessly for ingestible antennas.

5.7 CONCLUSION

The use of antennas in various biomedical applications in increasing day-by-day. The antennas are very much useful in diagnosing and detecting various diseases without much hassle. A lot of research has been done in the designing and use of WCE which gives clear high-resolution images of the internal body organs (like the highly convoluted small intestine), which otherwise was a very difficult task using classic endoscopic techniques. Antennas have also played a key role in the treatment of diseases like cancer using hyperthermia, where the tumor cells can be targeted and burned. This enhances the effectiveness of other therapies like chemotherapy and radiotherapy which are being given to cancer patients.

REFERENCES

[1] A. Rosen, M. A. Stuchly, and A. V. Vorst, "Applications of RF/microwaves in medicine," *IEEE Transactions on Microwave Theory and Techniques*, vol. 50, no. 3, pp. 963–974, 2002.

[2] A. Rosen and H. D. Rosen, "The role of engineering principles in the medical utilization of electromagnetic energies from kHz to visible light - examples," *Journal of Infrared, Millimeter, and Terahertz Waves*, vol. 30, no. 12, pp. 1374–1386, 2009.

[3] P. S. Hall and Y. Hao, "Antennas and propagation for body centric communications," *First European Conference on Antennas and Propagation, Nice*, pp. 1–7, 2006.
[4] E. Topsakal, "Antennas for medical applications: Ongoing research and future challenges," *International Conference on Electromagnetics in Advanced Applications*, Torino, pp. 890–893, 2009.
[5] P. Soontornpipit, C. M. Furse, and Y. C. Chung, "Design of implantable microstrip antenna for communication with medical implants," *IEEE Transactions on Microwave Theory and Techniques*, vol. 52, no. 8, pp. 1944–1951, 2004.
[6] G. Kiziltas, D. Psychoudakis, J. L. Volakis, and N. Kikuchi, "Topology design optimization of dielectric substrates for bandwidth improvement of a patch antenna," *IEEE Transactions on Antennas and Propagation*, vol. 51, no. 10, pp. 2732–2743, 2003.
[7] Y. Zhou, C. Chen and J. L. Volakis, "Dual band proximity-fed stacked patch antenna for tri-band GPS applications," *IEEE Transactions on Antennas and Propagation*, vol. 55, no. 1, pp. 220–223, 2007.
[8] Z. Tang, B. Smith, J. H. Schild, and P. H. Peckham, "Data transmission from an implantable biotelemeter by load-shift keying using circuit configuration modulator," *IEEE Transactions on Biomedical Engineering*, vol. 42, no. 5, pp. 524–528, 1995.
[9] P. Valdastri, A. Menciassi, A. Arena, C. Caccamo, and P. Dario, "An implantable telemetry platform system for in vivo monitoring of physiological parameters," *IEEE Transactions on Information Technology in Biomedicine*, vol. 8, no. 3, pp. 271–278, 2004.
[10] E. Y. Chow, M. M. Morris, and P. P. Irazoqui, "Implantable RF medical devices: the benefits of high-speed communication and much greater communication distances in biomedical applications," *IEEE Microwave Magazine*, vol. 14, no. 4, pp. 64–73, 2013.
[11] C. H. Durney and M. F. Iskander, "Antennas for medical applications" in *Antenna Handbook*, MA, Boston: Springer, 1993.
[12] M. R. Basar, F. Malek, K. M. Juni, M. S. Idris, M. Iskandar, and M. Saleh, "Ingestible wireless capsule technology: a review of development and future indication," *International Journal of Antennas and Propagation*, vol. 2012, Article ID 807165, 14 pages, 2012.
[13] T. Karacolak, A. Z. Hood, and E. Topsakal, "Design of a dual-band implantable antenna and development of skin mimicking gels for continuous glucose monitoring," *IEEE Transactions on Microwave Theory and Techniques*, vol. 56, no. 4, pp. 1001–1008, 2008.
[14] A. Kiourti and K. S. Nikita, "A review of implantable patch antennas for biomedical telemetry: Challenges and solutions [wireless corner]," *IEEE Antennas and Propagation Magazine*, vol. 54, no. 3, pp. 210–228, 2012.
[15] J. Kim and Y. Rahmat-Samii, "Implanted antennas inside a human body: simulations, designs, and characterizations," *IEEE Transactions on Microwave Theory and Techniques*, vol. 52, no. 8, pp. 1934–1943, 2004.
[16] C. J. Sanchez-Fernandez, O. Quevedo-Teruel, J. Requena-Carrion, L. Inclan-Sanchez, and E. Rajo-Iglesias, "Dual-band microstrip patch antenna based on short-circuited ring and spiral resonators for implantable medical devices," *IET Microwaves, Antennas & Propagation*, vol. 4, no. 8, pp. 1048–1055, 2010.
[17] H. Permana, Q. Fang and I. Cosic, "3-layer implantable microstrip antenna optimised for retinal prosthesis system in MICS band," *International Symposium on Bioelectronics and Bioinformations*, Suzhou, pp. 65–68, 2011.
[18] W-C. Liu, S-H. Chen, and C-M. Wu, "Implantable broadband circular stacked PIFA antenna for biotelemetry communication," *Journal of Electromagnetic Waves and Applications*, vol. 22, no. 13, pp. 1791–1800, 2008.
[19] J. Kim and Y. Rahmat-Samii, "Planar inverted-F antennas on implantable medical devices: Meandered type versus spiral type," *Microwave and Optical Technology Letters*, vol. 48, no. 3, pp. 567–572, 2006.

[20] P. Soontornpipit, C. M. Furse, and Y. C. Chung, "Miniaturized biocompatible microstrip antenna using genetic algorithm," *IEEE Transactions on Antennas and Propagation*, vol. 53, no. 6, pp. 1939–1945, 2005.

[21] A. Kiourti, M. Tsakalakis, and K. S. Nikita, "Parametric study and design of implantable PIFAs for wireless biotelemetry," *International Conference on Wireless Mobile Communication and Healthcare*, Berlin, Heidelberg: Springer, 2011.

[22] W.-C. Liu, F.-M. Yeh, and M. Ghavami, "Miniaturized implantable broadband antenna for biotelemetry communication," *Microwave and Optical Technology Letters*, vol. 50, no. 9, pp. 2407–2409, 2008.

[23] C.-M. Lee, T.-C. Yo, C.-H. Luo, C.-H. Tu, and Y.-Z. Juang, "Compact broadband stacked implantable antenna for biotelemetry with medical devices," *Electronics Letters*, vol. 43, no. 12, pp. 660–662, 2007.

[24] A. Kiourti, M. Christopoulou, and K. S. Nikita, "Performance of a novel miniature antenna implanted in the human head for wireless biotelemetry," *IEEE International Symposium on Antennas and Propagation*, Spokane, WA, pp. 392–395, 2011.

[25] S. A. Kumar and T. Shanmuganantham, "CPW fed dual V-shaped Implantable monopole antenna for biomedical applications," *IEEE International Conference on Computational Intelligence and Computing Research*, Coimbatore, pp. 1–4, 2012.

[26] Z. Duan, Y. Guo, R. Xue, M. Je, and D. Kwong, "Differentially fed dual-band implantable antenna for biomedical applications," *IEEE Transactions on Antennas and Propagation*, vol. 60, no. 12, pp. 5587–5595, 2012.

[27] F. Kong, C. Qi, H. Lee, G. D. Durgin, and M. Ghovanloo, "Antennas for intraoral tongue drive system at 2.4 GHz: Design, characterization, and comparison," *IEEE Transactions on Microwave Theory and Techniques*, vol. 66, no. 5, pp. 2546–2555, 2018.

[28] M. Zada and H. Yoo, "Miniaturized dual band antennas for intra-oral tongue drive system in the ISM bands 433 MHz and 915 MHz: Design, safety, and link budget considerations," *IEEE Transactions on Antennas and Propagation*, vol. 67, no. 9, pp. 5843–5852, 2019.

[29] M. Nachiappan and T. Azhagarsamy, "Design and development of dual-spiral antenna for implantable biomedical applications," *Biomedical Research*, vol. 28, no. 12, pp. 5237–5240, 2017.

[30] G. Sun, B. Muneer, Y. Li, and Q. Zhu, "Ultracompact implantable design with integrated wireless power transfer and RF transmission capabilities," *IEEE Transactions on Biomedical Circuits and Systems*, vol. 12, no. 2, pp. 281–291, 2018.

[31] H. Rajagopalan and Y. Rahmat-Samii, "Wireless medical telemetry characterization for ingestible capsule antenna designs," *IEEE Antennas and Wireless Propagation Letters*, vol. 11, pp. 1679–1682, 2012.

[32] F. El Hatmi, M. Grzeskowiak, S. Protat, and O. Picon, "Link budget of magnetic antennas for ingestible capsule at 40 MHz," *Progress In Electromagnetics Research*, vol. 134, pp. 111–131, 2013.

[33] S. H. Lee *et al.*, "A wideband spiral antenna for ingestible capsule endoscope systems: Experimental results in a human phantom and a pig," *IEEE Transactions on Biomedical Engineering*, vol. 58, no. 6, pp. 1734–1741, 2011.

[34] K. A. Psathas, A. Kiourti, and K. S. Nikita, "A novel conformal antenna for ingestible capsule endoscopy in the MedRadio band," *Progress In Electromagnetics Research Symposium Proceedings*, Stockholm, Sweden, pp. 1899–1902, 2013.

[35] P. Salonen, L. Sydanheimo, M. Keskilammi, and M. Kivikoski, "A small planar inverted-F antenna for wearable applications," *Digest of Papers. Third International Symposium on Wearable Computers*, San Francisco, CA, USA, pp. 95–100, 1999.

[36] P. Salonen and J. Rantanen, "A dual-band and wide-band antenna on flexible substrate for smart clothing," *27th Annual Conference of the IEEE Industrial Electronics Society*, Denver, CO, USA, vol. 1, pp. 125–130, 2001.

[37] J. C. G. Matthews, B. Pirollo, A. Tyler, and G. Pettitt, "Body wearable antennas for UHF/VHF," *Loughborough Antennas and Propagation Conference*, Loughborough, London, pp. 357–360, 2008.
[38] M. Klemm, I. Locher, and G. Troster, "A novel circularly polarized textile antenna for wearable applications," *34th European Microwave Conference*, Amsterdam, The Netherlands, pp. 137–140, 2004.
[39] C. A. Balanis, *Antenna Theory: Analysis and Design*, John Wiley & Sons, New York, 2016.
[40] C. Hertleer, H. Rogier, and L. V. Langenhove, "A textile antenna for protective clothing," *IET Seminar on Antennas and Propagation for Body-Centric Wireless Communications*, London, pp. 44–46, 2007.
[41] S. Zhu, L. Liu, and R. Langley, "Dual band body worn antenna," *Loughborough Antennas and Propagation Conference*, Loughborough, London, pp. 137–140, 2007.
[42] C. Hertleer, A. Tronquo, H. Rogier, L. Vallozzi, and L. Van Langenhove, "Aperture-coupled patch antenna for integration into wearable textile systems," *IEEE Antennas and Wireless Propagation Letters*, vol. 6, pp. 392–395, 2007.
[43] G. Kumar and K. P. Ray, *Broadband Microstrip Antennas*, Artech House, Boston, London, 2003.
[44] H. H. Kuhn, A. D. Child, and W. C. Kimbrell, "Toward real applications of conductive polymers," *Synthetic Metals*, vol. 71, no. 1-3, pp. 2139–2142, 1995.
[45] I. Locher, M. Klemm, T. Kirstein, and G. Trster, "Design and characterization of purely textile patch antennas," *IEEE Transactions on Advanced Packaging*, vol. 29, no. 4, pp. 777–788, 2006.
[46] C. Hertleer, H. Rogier, L. Vallozzi, and F. Declercq, "A textile antenna based on high-performance fabrics," *The Second European Conference on Antennas and Propagation*, Edinburgh, pp. 1–5, 2007.
[47] M. Klemm and G. Troster, "Textile UWB antenna for on-body communications," *First European Conference on Antennas and Propagation*, Nice, pp. 1–4, 2006.
[48] J. G. Santas, A. Alomainy, and Y. Hao, "Textile antennas for on-body communications: Techniques and properties," *The Second European Conference on Antennas and Propagation*, Edinburgh, pp. 1–4, 2007.
[49] P. Salonen, J. Kim, and Y. Rahmat-Samii, "Dual-band E-shaped patch wearable textile antenna," *IEEE Antennas and Propagation Society International Symposium*, Washington, DC, vol. 1A, pp. 466–469, 2005.
[50] IEEE standards for safety levels with request to human exposure to radiofrequency electromagnetic fields, 3 kHz to 300 GHz, IEEE Std. C95.1. 1999.
[51] A. Ahlbom *et al.*, "Guidelines for limiting exposure to time-varying electric, magnetic, and electromagnetic fields (up to 300 GHz)," *Health Physics*, vol. 74, no. 4, pp. 494–521, 1998.
[52] Y. Rahmat-Samii, "Wearable and implantable antennas in body-centric communications," *The Second European Conference on Antennas and Propagation*, Edinburgh, pp. 1–5, 2007.
[53] K. Ito, "Recent small antennas for medical applications," *International Workshop on Antenna Technology: Small Antennas and Novel Metamaterials*, Chiba, pp. 1–4, 2008.
[54] K. Ito, K. Saito, and M. Takahashi, "Small antennas for medical applications," *International Workshop on Antenna Technology: Small and Smart Antennas Metamaterials and Applications*, Cambridge, pp. 116–119, 2007.

6 Wearable Sensors for Monitoring Exercise and Fatigue Estimation in Rehabilitation

Maria J. Pinto-Bernal[1], Andres Aguirre[2], Carlos A. Cifuentes[3], and Marcela Munera[4]
[1-4]Department of Biomedical Engineering, Colombian School of Engineering Julio Garavito, AK 45 #205-59, Bogotá, Colombia.

CONTENTS

6.1 Introduction 84
6.2 Physical Exercise in Rehabilitation 85
 6.2.1 Health-Related Physical Components 86
 6.2.2 Exercise Restraint 87
6.3 Fatigue 87
 6.3.1 Subjective Scales 89
 6.3.2 Physiological Parameters 89
 6.3.3 Exercise Performance 89
6.4 Instruments for Measuring Fatigue 89
 6.4.1 Borg Scale 90
 6.4.2 Oxygen Uptake 90
 6.4.3 Heart Rate 91
 6.4.4 Blood Lactate Level 91
 6.4.5 Surface Electromyography 92
 6.4.6 Motion Analysis 92
 6.4.7 Inertial Sensors 93
6.5 Experimental Studies 94
 6.5.1 Recruiting Criteria 94
 6.5.2 Aerobic Study 94
  6.5.2.1 Experimental Aerobic Procedure 94
  6.5.2.2 Results of the Aerobic Study 96
 6.5.3 Anaerobic Study 98
  6.5.3.1 Experimental Anaerobic Procedure 98
  6.5.3.2 Results of the Anaerobic Study 99

6.6 Discussion 102
6.7 Conclusions 103
References 104

6.1 INTRODUCTION

Physical exercise has become a fundamental part of different rehabilitation environments, as it improves patients' quality of life [67]. In this context, rehabilitation seeks to improve the physical capacity of the patient through aerobic or anaerobic exercises. However, the intensity of these exercises must be controlled. Overtrained patients experiment with high states of fatigue that can affect their rehabilitation and health [15]. In order to adjust these intensities, measurement of physiological parameters, subjective scales, and exercise performance have been implemented. This chapter is focused on both, the importance of physical exercise in rehabilitation along with the exercise restriction to avoid fatigue, and strategies for monitoring based on wearable sensors with huge potential for estimating fatigue levels.

According to the American Health Association (AHA), physical exercise is one of the main components of improving people's health and decreasing morbidity and mortality levels [30]. Physical exercise seeks to improve the person's physical capacity according to age, weight, and pathologies. Physical exercise and physical capacity have become a fundamental part of different areas of rehabilitation, such as cardiac rehabilitation, oncological rehabilitation, and neuromuscular rehabilitation.

Several methods have been explored to monitor the patients' fatigue state to supervise the exercise intensity during therapies and the patients' fatigue state. Fatigue has generally been defined as a subjective state of tiredness or exhaustion and the reduction of capacity for regular activity [1]. Additionally, fatigue is defined as the inability of the muscles to maintain the required level of strength during exercises. It can also result in the deterioration of health in the long term, including Work-Related Musculoskeletal Disorders (WMSDs) [10], chronic fatigue syndrome [5] and compromised immune function [50]. Therefore, fatigue is a common concern among people who participate in physical activities based on training or rehabilitation [1].

The human body exhibits physical fatigue in several ways. Thus, researchers have developed several methods to measure fatigue [1]. Current occupational fatigue assessments rely on subjective measurement scales, as questionnaires and self-perceived exertion scales [5, 52]. However, specific fatigue symptoms may vary depending on existing pathologies, environmental factors, and physical condition. Therefore, subjective measurements of fatigue often need to be adapted to the environment and the patient. In order to overcome these limitations, measurements of physiological parameters and exercise performance have been considered.

This chapter aims to present strategies for estimating performance-related fatigue in aerobic and anaerobic exercises using wearable sensors. In order to do so, it is necessary to understand the relevance of physical exercise, as well as the definition and importance of fatigue and its measurement strategies. The primary outcomes showed that the use of wearable sensors would measure and indicate the fatigue reflected in spatiotemporal and kinematics parameters during the execution of aerobic and anaerobic exercises.

This chapter is organized in seven thematic sections, addressing relevant aspects regarding fatigue measure and essential aspects covering physical exercise in rehabilitation settings.

Section 6.2 addresses the importance of physical exercises and its modulation in rehabilitation programs, paying particular attention to anaerobic and aerobic exercise.

Section 6.3 begins with the definition of fatigue, its classification, and a definition of muscle fatigue. This is followed by three strategies used in fatigue estimation.

Section 6.4 presents the most commonly used measures used in the three strategies reported in Section 6.3 for fatigue estimation.

Section 6.5 addresses two experimental studies in both aerobic and anaerobic exercises, which are based on measuring fatigue through performance decrease in physical exercises.

Section 6.6 discusses the fatigue measures in the decrease of performance and the outcomes obtained during the studies carried out.

Finally, Section 6.7 presents the conclusions, some recommendations for future works in this field and the challenges of fatigue estimation in the rehabilitation context.

6.2 PHYSICAL EXERCISE IN REHABILITATION

Physical Exercise (PE) is understood as any activity that requires contracting muscles and more energy expenditure than a resting state [67]. Performing physical activity provides numerous benefits to people's health, such as the improvement of the cardiorespiratory system and the development of muscular groups, which are essential for daily life tasks [61]. Besides, the Word Health Organization (WHO) highly recommends PE to prevent and treat many chronic diseases, such as cardiovascular diseases, cancer, stroke, and diabetes [78].

Several rehabilitation programs have incorporated PE in their therapies; for example, in (i) cardiac rehabilitation, to increase the patient's cardiovascular performance [19, 32, 54]; (ii) oncology rehabilitation, to ease the effects of pathological fatigue [18, 65], which is a symptom normally presented in patients with cancer [46] that make them get tired easily when performing daily life activities [20]; (iii) neuromuscular rehabilitation, to recover mobility of limbs, by retraining and fixing the affected neural paths [15, 38, 68]; (iv) pulmonary rehabilitation, to raise the pulmonary capacity of the patients [26, 66]; and (v) musculoskeletal rehabilitation, to recover joint mobility and muscular strength after surgery [22, 23]. This information is summarized in Table 6.1.

The inadequate use of PE can lead to extreme physical or physiological conditions that can result in health complications, especially if previous heart or pulmonary disease is present [41]. Therefore, several considerations need to be taken into account when implementing PE in rehabilitation and designing exercises according to each individual's needs and conditions [53].

TABLE 6.1
Physical Exercise Objectives in Rehabilitation Programs

Rehabilitation Program	Physical Exercise Goal
Cardiac	Improve the cardiac system capability
Oncology	Mitigate the effects of pathological fatigue
Neuromuscular	Retrain the affected movement neural paths
Pulmonary	Improve the respiratory system capability
Musculoskeletal	Recover joint strength after surgery

6.2.1 Health-Related Physical Components

PE in rehabilitation is focused on developing health-related physical components, which are the necessary body elements for having a good quality of life. These physical components can be classified into four individual groups (Table 6.2) [49]: (i) body composition contemplates the distribution of different tissues in the body (fats, water, muscle, and bone) and it is worked with diet and exercise [49]; (ii) musculoskeletal refers to the power, flexibility, resistance and strength of the muscles and joints, trained by performing endurance and stretching activities with external loads or bodyweight [71]; (iii) aerobic capability is related to the ability of the cardiac and respiratory systems to provide oxygen for creating energy (also known as the cardiorespiratory group), and developed by means of long-duration activities (between 20 to 60 minutes) with low intensity [72]; and (iv) anaerobic capability is the body's capacity to create energy without using oxygen for short-duration movements with high intensity [71]. It is worth mentioning that anaerobic capability was not an essential skill for a healthy life in the beginning. Nevertheless, several studies have shown that it is essential for sudden daily life movements, and now its development is included in the AHA manual [21, 70, 73].

Due to the diversity of exercises, it is possible to generate a training plan that adapts to the patient's unique conditions (e.g., age, weight, medication, existing

TABLE 6.2
Health-Related Physical Components Groups

Group	Meaning	Training Method
Body composition	Tissue distribution	Diet and general exercise
Musculoskeletal	Muscle strength and flexibility	Endurance and stretching exercise
Aerobic capability	Create energy with oxygen	Soft activities with long duration
Anaerobic capability	Create energy without oxygen	Hard activities with short duration

pathologies, and injuries). For example, patients who are overweight are advised to train with extracorporeal loads (for the musculoskeletal group) or with an ergometer (for the aerobic and anaerobic groups), because it is easier and safer for them than moving their body mass [34]. Furthermore, studies have shown that better rehabilitation results are obtained when elderly patients with osteoporosis use weight-bearing in their therapies because these types of exercises allow them to reach the highest mechanical load on bones [63]. In contrast, it is suggested that patients with cancer and average weight, perform exercise that requires to move the body weight, such as: climbing upstairs, walking on a treadmill or sitting and standing up, because these motions reflect the daily activities that they cannot handle [51, 65, 76].

6.2.2 Exercise Restraint

One technique used to regulate the exercise intensity in training is the Metabolic Equivalent (MET). This unit represents the relationship between the rate of energy spent on physical activity and the rate of energy spent at rest [3]. In other words, it is defined as the caloric consumption of an active individual compared to the resting basal metabolic rate. This information is useful for prescribing exercise intensity, as well as to identify the functional capacity of the patient. For that, this method needs to estimate the amount of energy that each person uses to perform a specific activity. Its requirement makes it complex to estimate the exact MET value, because it depends on the subject's characteristics (e.g., metabolism and weight) and requires complex instrumentation [61]. Therefore, several studies have been dedicated to generalize the MET values of different activities, based on measurements from healthy study subjects [61]. This generalization allows the clinical staff to select the activities for the training plan [4] and provides a practical, easy way to quantify the energy cost. However, this way of measuring exercise intensity has been criticized because it does not consider that some people have different chronic diseases or have a higher level of fitness than others; therefore, it does not provide a real-time patient condition [60].

Thus, aiming to solve this issue, one of the most explored methods consists of estimating the fatigue perceived by the patient [6].

6.3 FATIGUE

Fatigue has been considered as a subjective experience. Great efforts have been made to conceptualize it as a subjective state of sleepiness, tiredness, or exhaustion of normal activity capacity [1]. Fatigue is a term used to describe a decrease in physical performance associated with an increase in the real/perceived difficulty of a task or exercise [5]. The level of human fatigue is correlated with performance indicators such as work productivity, performance, athletic results, injuries, mistakes, and accidents.

There are many different fatigue classification methods. According to its duration, fatigue can be classified into acute and chronic fatigue. Acute fatigue results from short-term sleep loss or short periods of substantial physical or mental work. The effects of acute fatigue are of short duration and usually can be reversed by sleep and relaxation [43]. Chronic fatigue syndrome is a constant, severe state of tiredness that is not relieved by rest. The symptoms of chronic fatigue syndrome are similar to the flu, last longer than 6 months, and interfere with certain activities. The exact cause of this syndrome is still unknown. On the other hand, fatigue can also be classified as mental fatigue, which refers to the cognitive or perceptual aspects of fatigue, and physical fatigue, which refers to the performance of the motor system [10].

Muscle fatigue is a transient and recoverable reduction in the force or power production in response to contractile activity. It is a symptom that makes it harder to move as normal [69]. It can originate at different motor pathway levels and is usually divided into central and peripheral components. Peripheral fatigue refers to exercise-induced processes that lead to a reduction in force production occurring at distal to the neuromuscular junction. Central fatigue refers to more centralized processes and can be defined as a progressive exercise-induced failure of voluntary activation of the muscle, which is not associated with the same reduction of maximum force obtained by stimulation [70]. Muscle fatigue is a commonly experienced phenomenon where people always feel tired and lack energy, resulting in limited performance and other strenuous or prolonged daily activities. Also, some people experience a dull aching in the muscle. It also increases and restricts daily life.

Therefore, it is essential to understand the implications and consequences of fatigue. For instance, it can result in the deterioration of health in the long term, including work-related musculoskeletal disorders, chronic fatigue syndrome, and compromised immune function [50]. Besides, fatigue is a common symptom associated with a wide range of chronic diseases such as cancer, multiple sclerosis, cardiovascular, Parkinson, as well as fibromyalgia symptoms [7, 12, 48].

In this context, fatigue plays an essential role in Physical Rehabilitation (PR). The WHO Organization defines PR as an active process to achieve a full recovery or, if full recovery is not possible, to reach optimal physical, mental, and social potential to integrate people appropriately into society [78]. As a comprehensive strategy, PR has two approaches:

1. Improve cognitive aspects related to the cognition processes that include perception, language, and motivation.
2. Improve physical aspects of patients such as aerobic and anaerobic capabilities, cardiovascular functioning, gait patterns during physical activity and muscle.

These approaches are important to assess the patient's long-term performance and achieve a full recovery and a successful rehabilitative process. Notwithstanding this, fatigue is prevalent worrying among people who engage in physical activities based on rehabilitation [9]. Hence, the ability to quantify fatigue allows a measure of severity and the subsequent identification of health and safety issues, enabling the regulation of the intensity of the physical exercise in the rehabilitation process and its subjective nature [1]. Regarding the importance of fatigue monitoring, different strategies have been developed in order to measure fatigue [9]. These strategies include subjective scales of fatigue perception, physiological parameters, and exercise performance.

6.3.1 Subjective Scales

The subjective scales of fatigue perception are ordinal numerical scales in which each represents a level of fatigue in such a way that the lower number represents a state of absence of fatigue, and the higher number represents a state of extreme fatigue. In extreme fatigue, the person does not feel able to carry out the physical exercise [80]. According to the environment where fatigue is estimated, different scales of perception are used and even modified according to their application [52]. One of the most implemented is the Borg Rating of Perceived Exertion (RPE) scale. Several studies have illustrated that perception scales present subjectivity and differences concerning other methods of estimation of fatigue, such as physiological parameters, thus leading to a decrease in the reliability of this method [62].

6.3.2 Physiological Parameters

Physiological parameters determine a person's physiological state, as they indicate the body's internal functioning [5]. One of the applications is the indirect estimation of fatigue. The parameters most related are heart rate, oxygen consumption, blood pressure, respiratory rate, and blood lactate level [36, 45, 50, 79]. According to the type of exercise performed, these parameters may present different behaviors, making it difficult to relate to the level of tiredness, and some even present difficulties when monitoring in real-time; therefore, researchers are looking for new estimation strategies [31].

6.3.3 Exercise Performance

The decrease in exercise performance has a directly proportional relationship with the increase in fatigue [31]. Therefore, methods for monitoring fatigue through exercise performance have been implemented. However, their evaluation depends heavily on the type of exercise used [39]. The parameters and characteristics to be evaluated depend on each exercise and must be sure to avoid errors or uncertainties in the measurements. For example, if an exercise is performed on a treadmill, the commonly evaluated parameters are the cadence, the width, and length of step, the duration of each gait phase, among others [55]. The evaluation of exercise can be performed in different ways using ambulatory sensors (e.g., inertial sensors and electromyography) and non-ambulatory sensors (e.g., motion analysis system).

6.4 INSTRUMENTS FOR MEASURING FATIGUE

This section presents the most commonly used fatigue measurement instruments based on the three different strategies explained above. It is important to note that so far, there is not a method established to measure fatigue. It is leading to a slow assessment of the reliability, validity, and usefulness of fatigue measures for the physician and the researcher, given the few reviews from which to draw such information.

6.4.1 Borg Scale

The Borg Rating of Perceived Exertion (RPE) scale is a tool for measuring an individual's effort and exertion, breathlessness and fatigue during physical work and is highly relevant for occupational health and safety practice.

The scale is a simple numerical list. It starts with "no feeling of exertion", which rates a 6, and ends with "very, very hard", which rates a 20. The scale takes seconds to complete and can be done by a researcher or self-administered and used on a single occasion or multiple times.

During the activity, participants are asked to rate their exertion on the scale, combining all sensation and feeling of physical stress and fatigue. They are told to disregard any one factor such as leg pain or shortness of breath but to try to focus on the whole feeling of exertion. This number indicates the intensity of activity, allowing the participant to speed up or slow down movements [74].

Borg also developed the Borg CR10, a Category-Ratio (CR) scale anchored at the number 10, representing an extreme intensity of activity. It is a general method for measuring most kinds of perceptions and experiences, including pain and also perceived exertion. Figure 6.1 illustrates the representation of the RPE and Borg CR10.

6.4.2 Oxygen Uptake

The oxygen uptake (VO_2, normally measured in mLO_2/min/kg), is considered as one of the best ways to quantify the patient's fatigue, because of its linear relationship with the energy cost [57]. In fact, the VO_2 can be changed easily to MET units implementing Equation 6.1 [35]. However, the VO_2 measurement requires complex instrumentation, which makes it impractical for rehabilitation therapies, and it is

Borg scale	Borg CR10	Representation
6	0	No exertion
7		
8	1	Very very low exertion
9		
10	2	Very low exertion
11		
12	3	Low exertion
13		
14	4	Quite moderate exertion
15	5	Somewhat moderate exertion
16	6	Moderate exertion
17	7	High exertion
18	8	Very high exertion
19	9	Very very high exertion
20	10	Maximum fatigue level

FIGURE 6.1 Borg scale table.

normally used for research scenarios [35]. Besides, it requires a changeable signal which in turn requires a stabilization time [35].

$$1(MET) = 3.5(mLO_2/\text{min}/kg) \tag{6.1}$$

6.4.3 Heart Rate

The heart rate is one of the most commonly used physiological parameters to control fatigue, owing to its facility of measuring and the linear relationship that it presents with the VO_2 [17]. In general, this methodology consists of monitoring the heart rate reserve, which is the difference between the Maximum Heart Rate (MHR) and the Resting Heart Rate (RHR) [70]. The MHR can be estimated using a stress test, a clinical test that assesses the body's physiological behavior during different exercises [37]. Nevertheless, there are more practical ways that consider some subject's characteristics (e.g., age and gender) to get an approximation. One of the most implemented is Tanaka's formula that uses the user's age (in years) and is shown in Equation 6.2 [14].

$$MHR = 206.9 - (0.67 * AGE) \tag{6.2}$$

In order to show an example, it is supposed a 21-year-old person (MHR = 193 approximately, using Equation 6.2) with an RHR of 80 *BPM*, which means that his Heart Rate Reserve (HRR) is equal to 113 *BPM*. Therefore, if the subject presents a heart rate of 150 *BPM*, this represents the 62% of his HRR. This process can be seen in Equation 6.3, where HRR% is the percentage of the subject's HRR and HR is the current heart rate value.

$$HRR\% = \frac{100}{HRR} * (HR - RHR) \tag{6.3}$$

It is considered that physical training which requires a HRR% between 60 to 80% is high intensity, and depending on the rehabilitation goal and the patient conditions, this state should be avoided [70]. The heart rate gives a direct measurement of the subject. However, its interpretation requires some assumptions based on healthy people and does not consider other features that could affect the heart rate (e.g., medication and pathologies) [14]. Hence, this method has been criticized for fatigue management in physical rehabilitation.

6.4.4 Blood Lactate Level

Lactate is a biochemical indicator of decreased organ perfusion, decreased oxygen delivery or extraction, and end-organ anaerobic glycolysis [33]. The glycolysis is the metabolic pathway that uses glucose for creating pyruvate, which can be used by the aerobic or anaerobic metabolism to create energy. When the exercise is quite intense, all pyruvate cannot be processed by the aerobic way. Therefore, it is converted in lactate and accumulated in blood by the anaerobic metabolism to get more energy and harness the amount of pyruvate produced [33]. The blood lactate level provides a direct measurement of the subject exertion during the exercise. Therefore, the lactate threshold is a useful measure of determining exercise intensity for the training or rehabilitation context. However, it requires to get a blood sample and a specialized instrument, which is not always easy to use during physical therapies [59]. Besides, it is a parameter highly dependent on aerobic or anaerobic exercise and the user's metabolism. Hence, it is required to constantly monitorize this parameter to get a good interpretation [33, 59].

Aerobic Threshold: The aerobic threshold is defined as the exercise intensity at which the blood lactate concentration rises above rest levels. It is the exercise intensity at which aerobic energy pathways start to operate, considered to be around 65–85% of an individual's maximum heart rate [27].

Anaerobic Threshold: The anaerobic threshold is defined as the exercise intensity at which the blood lactate concentration is no longer linearly related to exercise intensity, but increases with both exercise intensity and duration [25].

6.4.5 Surface Electromyography

Surface Electromyography (EMG) is another ambulatory system, which consists of measuring the electrical activity generated during muscle contraction and relaxation [47]. The function is to attach electrodes to the muscles in order to register electrical potentials [56]. These potentials are directly related to muscular strength, which allows to estimate the effort and evaluate the performance of the exercise [77]. Nevertheless, these electrical signals are affected by the impedance of the skin and the electrodes' location. Therefore, an initial normalization process is required to avoid these problems leading to low adaptability [13, 44].

In recent years, different studies have established EMGs as a non-invasive alternative for estimating muscle fatigue [1, 13]. The electrical activity signal presents changes in its frequency and morphology, i.e., it presents a decrease in its amplitude and an increase in its duration [8, 11, 13].

6.4.6 Motion Analysis

The motion analysis system is based on the use of infrared cameras to estimate the position of reflective markers in order to segment an object or an individual, and measure variables such as position and orientation [58]. These systems can measure a large number of kinematic parameters and, according to the kinematic model, can implement estimated specific characteristics of each movement or exercise, which has led to its high applicability in these areas [29].

Motion analysis is widely used in fatigue estimation due to its high accuracy and robustness in the measurement of kinematic parameters. Muscular fatigue affects movement and gait characteristics as impaired motor control and postural instability [45]. The aim of using these devices is to quantify and measure these different parameters. Likewise, identify when an event exists outside the typical pattern to help in the rehabilitation process and the performance of the activities [75]. However, these devices present certain limitations in terms of their sophisticated instrumentation, low adaptability in different environments, and their high cost [24].

6.4.7 Inertial Sensors

The most used ambulatory systems are the inertial sensors. Inertial sensors are gaining increasing popularity in human motion analysis as components of wearable sensor systems that provide motion data directly, without the use of external sources or devices.

The Inertial Measurement Unit (IMU) is essentially the combination of two components: accelerometers and gyroscopes; with them, this device can measure gravitational force, speed, and orientation. Moreover, with these parameters, it is possible to make estimations of the motion analysis [16], gait phases [40], as well as temporal space parameters [2]. It is instrumental to assess the performance of some activity, and with this, it is possible to identify the level of fatigue of the person. It should be noted that IMUs can incorporate magnetometers to obtain a better estimate of orientation, using fusion sensor techniques.

Accelerometers are the most widely used option if an outpatient motion or gait analysis is required; these have certain advantages, such as miniaturization, high mobility, low cost, and power. However, their use carries several factors, such as the need to perform gravity compensations according to the acceleration calculation. The more computational load is required in the post-processing stage, there is an occurrence of drift error in position data. It is necessary to calibrate the system to locate the sensors in the required segment accurately [40].

Gyroscopes are angular velocity sensors; this velocity is a factor whose signal is not influenced by the vibrations (e.g., the vibrations that occur at the moment of hitting the heel); additionally, this variable is not affected by the force of gravity. In the output of a gyroscope are obtained periodic results whose patterns are repeated during a periodic interval of exercise, such as the gait cycle, jumping, riding a bicycle, sitting down and standing up [42].

To provide 3D motion analysis, the inertial units usually incorporate three perpendicular accelerometers and three gyroscopes, represented as the x, y, and z axes of the unit. These sensors allow studying one movement regardless of its direction by estimating the magnitude of these measurements. This magnitude estimation can be seen in Equation 6.4, where MAG represents the magnitude of the signal.

$$MAG = \sqrt{x^2 + y^2 + z^2} \tag{6.4}$$

Taking into account the techniques presented, the next section describes the experimental studies that were carried out. Aiming to analyze and evaluate the fatigue in aerobic and anaerobic exercises.

6.5 EXPERIMENTAL STUDIES

This section presents, in the first place, the criteria implemented for recruiting volunteers; subsequently, it describes the experimental studies carried out for fatigue estimation in aerobic and anaerobic exercises. Both exercises were implemented due to differences in their performance and energy generation. Aerobic exercise produces energy using a continuous supply of oxygen to sustain the current activity level without needing additional energy from another source. Whereas, anaerobic exercise prompts the body to demand more energy than the aerobic system can produce [27].

6.5.1 Recruiting Criteria

Each subject voluntarily agreed to participate in these experiments and signed the corresponding informed consent. Volunteers were selected according to the inclusion and exclusion criteria described below.

Inclusion Criteria: Healthy adult subjects between 18 to 30 years old who perform regular physical activity and have no contraindications for exercise. Besides, the subjects did not have any prostheses or orthosis in their lower or upper limbs.

Exclusion Criteria: Volunteers with any visual, auditory, or cognitive impairments that prevent the correct understanding of the activity were not part of this study. Likewise, the volunteer must not present injuries, pain, or surgeries in the knee, ankle, or hip. On the other hand, the volunteer must not be pregnant. Finally, the volunteer must not present any fatigue that may affect his performance, which was assessed by mean of the "multidimensional fatigue inventory", which is a 20-item questionnaire to estimate five different types of fatigue: general fatigue, physical fatigue, mental fatigue, reduced motivation, and reduced activity [64].

6.5.2 Aerobic Study

An aerobic study is conducted to assess if the physical fatigue can be measured with wearable sensors such as inertial measurement units. The study was executed on a male volunteer with the following characteristics: age: 22 years old, weight: 76.9 kg, and height: 1.86 cm.

6.5.2.1 Experimental Aerobic Procedure

The volunteer was first instructed to perform three 10 m tests at a self-selected speed to determine their average overground speed, which was successively set on a treadmill. The participant was equipped with five Shimmer3 (Shimmer, Ireland) IMU units, which are necessary to measure the spatiotemporal and kinematic parameters. Four units were configured to obtain EMG signals in four muscles (tibialis anterior, rectus femoris, biceps femoris, and gastrocnemius) with a sampling rate of 512 Hz. Two are located on the outer lateral part of the thighs, and two on the calves' outer side with elastic bands. The last unit was configured as an inertial measurement unit with a sample rate of 128 Hz. The IMU was placed on instep of the participant's dominant foot (in this case, the left one) with an elastic band. The experimental setup described here is illustrated in Figure 6.2.

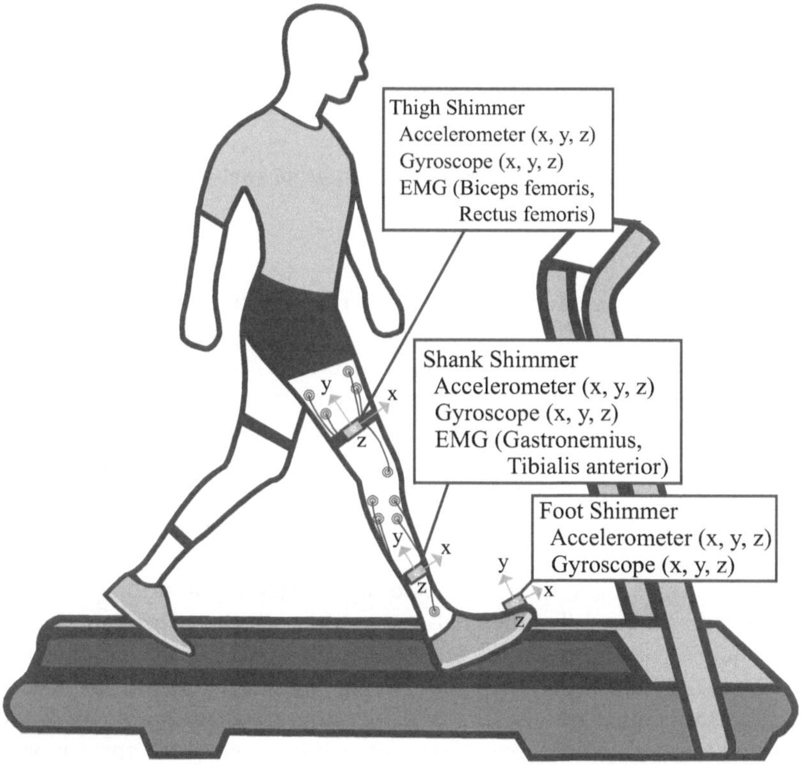

FIGURE 6.2 Experimental setup. Participant was instrumented on their dominant side with an IMU placed on the dorsal side of their foot. Likewise, with four more IMUs located on each thigh and shank and with different electrodes located on the tibialis anterior, rectus femoris, biceps femoris, and gastrocnemius.

The volunteer was asked to participate in a short study consisting of one session with four stages. Each stage had the same four exercises: high knees, jumping jacks, squats, and short runs. The difference between the steps was the duration of each task, which was progressively increasing, i.e., the corresponding time of each exercise was 30 s (first step), 45 s (second step), 60 s (third step), and 75 s (fourth step).

In order to assess the fatigue, at the end of each stage, four parameters were measured: (i) Blood lactate level, (ii) a perceptive fatigue scale, the Borg CR10, both variables give and an indication of the fatigue level, (iii) EMG signals, and (iv) spatiotemporal parameters. Regarding the measurement of blood lactate, a blood sample was taken from the participant's earlobe with a lancet. The blood was collected with a new test strip, and finally, the strip was inserted into the Lactate Pro2 (Arkray, Japan) to measure the blood lactate level. On the other hand, the Borg CR10 scale was obtained by asking the volunteer how tired he felt according to the scale (Figure 6.1). We indicated to the participant that they should only concentrate on the sensation of total effort and not on the shortness of breath or muscle pain.

Concerning the measurement of the last two parameters, the participant was then asked to walk for at least 180 s on the already configured treadmill at a zero-degree inclination. Data acquisition only started once the self-selected speed was reached. The treadmill speed was only reduced after all data were acquired to prevent data capture during the transient state.

The entire experiment, including donning/doffing times related to instrumentation procedures, exercises, and walking tasks, was completed in 60 min.

6.5.2.2 Results of the Aerobic Study

According to the measurements considered during the study, some essential aspects are worthy of mention. In the first place, the performance of the session was successfully measured using the sensors previously described. As illustrated in Figure 6.3, a sample data of the muscular activity behavior in one gait cycle is presented. It should be noted that it was necessary to segment the gait cycle each time the toe-off phase occurred. The graph shows the muscular activity measured on the participant's left gastrocnemius muscle during the initial and final step in the session in one gait cycle. The muscular activity registered a significant decrease in the activation of electrical activity at the end-stage of the session.

In the same way, the muscle presented high variability at the beginning of the initial session, and the end of the final-step session, which can be associated with a delay in muscle activation. On the other hand, the time of the gait cycle increased in the final step, which may indicate that the volunteer lowered his cadence. It is essential to mention that this behavior was observed for both legs in the following measured muscles: tibialis anterior, rectus femoris, biceps femoris, and gastrocnemius.

It is essential to underline that concerning the results (A), (B), (D), (E), and (F) of Figure 6.4, the values were calculated using Equation 6.5. The test number zero was taken as a reference, since it was considered that the volunteer did not have fatigue, which was corroborated with the Borg CR10 scale and the blood lactate. It was carried out to analyze the behavior of these parameters more precisely when the

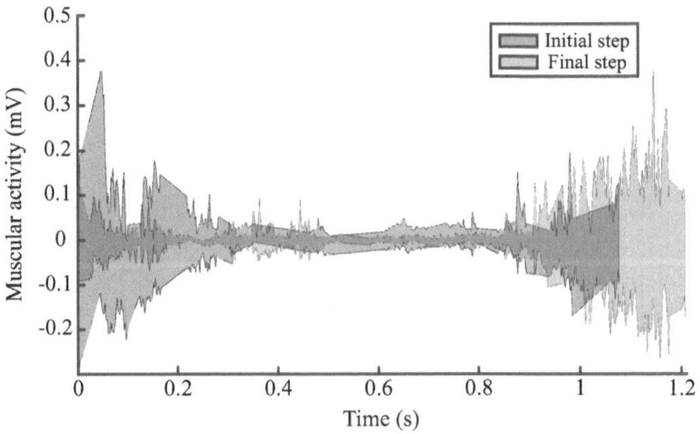

FIGURE 6.3 Muscular activity on the left gastrocnemius muscle in one gait cycle.

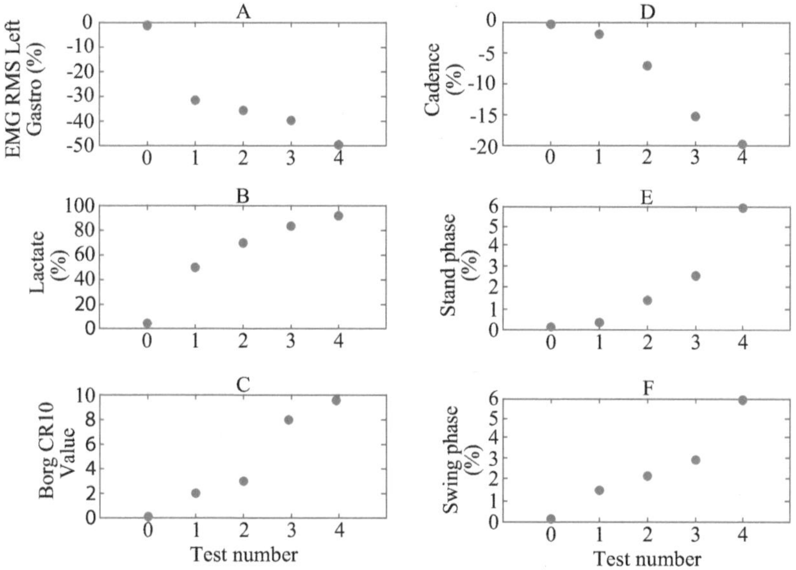

FIGURE 6.4 Participant's data registered during the session. (A) EMG RMS, (B) lactacte, (C) Borg CR10, (D) cadence, (E) stance phase, and (F) swing phase.

level of fatigue increases. Furthermore, the first three events (A), (B), and (C) were used as indicators of fatigue reference to analyze the behavior of the spatiotemporal parameters.

$$X_i = \left(\frac{X_i - X_{reference}}{X_i} \right) * 100\% \quad (6.5)$$

In this way, the behavior of muscular activity during the therapy session was analyzed. To this end, the mean of the electrical activity (RMS) was calculated through a window size of 100 miliseconds. The first window was used as a reference to calculate the change in the other moments. Figure 6.4 (A) illustrates this behavior in percentage throughout the session. The general conduct of the data recorded during the study and the effects of the fatigue over these parameters are illustrated in the same Figure 6.4. Plot (B) shows the lactate, and the Borg CR10 values requested during the session are plotted in diagram (C). Plots (D), (E), and (F) represent the spatiotemporal parameters (cadence, swing, and stance phase) behavior in percentage throughout the session. In order to obtain the spatiotemporal parameters, the gyroscope and accelerometer outputs were first treated with a median filter to eliminate atypical data values, and a second-order low-pass filter Butterworth (cut-off frequencies were defined according to the Fourier transformation) using MATLAB® software (The MathWorks, Inc., USA). Then, inertial signals were partitioned into each gait cycle, for that each toe-off phase was identified. Finally, the partitioned data of each gait

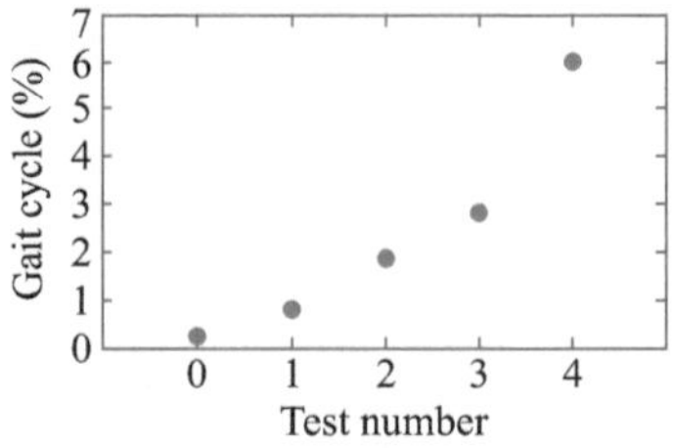

FIGURE 6.5 Increase in gait cycle at each stage in percentage.

event were time-normalized, and means of the obtained dataset were used to find the spatiotemporal parameters.

It can be observed that first the volunteer presents fatigue according to the blood lactate parameter, a low level in most parameters, as well as the self-perception of the fatigue estimated with Borg CR10. However, once the volunteer begins to present fatigue, the data recorded similarly reflect the increase as the blood lactate and the space-time change with an increasing rate. Nevertheless, the cadence presented a similar behavior, decreasing rate, and the RMS obtained. It means that the following variables: Lactate, Borg scale, gait cycle phases (swing and stand) are directly proportional, whereas the cadence and RMS are inversely proportional.

On the other hand, the percentage of the gait cycle in each stage concerning the initial stage was calculated to corroborate that the decrease in the cadence is due to an increase in the gait cycle, as shown in the behavior in both gait phases. As illustrated in Figure 6.5, there is an increment in the consecutive gait cycle as the volunteer began to present fatigue. The maximum increase in the gait cycle occurred in the last stage with an increase of 6.14%.

Based on the information that the sensors (IMUs) can record during each stage, it was possible to monitor and analyze the volunteer's performance throughout the aerobic exercise. Likewise, it was possible to note how fatigue is reflected in the exercise decrease performance.

6.5.3 Anaerobic Study

Aiming to show the implementation of IMU measurements in anaerobic exercises for estimating fatigue, this section of the chapter centers on presenting the results obtained in a study carried out with a healthy male volunteer (age: 23 years, weight: 68 Kg and height: 174 cm) who ride on a cycle ergometer during five minutes. Considering that he is a healthy subject, the maximum heart rate can be obtained with the Tanaka's formula (equation 6.2, 191 BPM approximately).

6.5.3.1 Experimental Anaerobic Procedure

The following procedure is based on one high-intensity training implemented in cardiac rehabilitation [28]. First, the volunteer was instructed in a 5-minute warm-up, composed of stretching activities focused on the lower limbs. Afterwards, the ergometer was configured in order for the volunteer to be able to extend the knees completely in the extension part of the movement and feel comfortable at riding.

The subject performed a cycle ergometer test, split into 10 training intervals and 10 resting intervals, one followed by the other, starting with one training interval and each one with a duration of 15 seconds. During the training intervals, the volunteer was asked to ride as fast as possible. On the other hand, during the resting intervals, he rode at a comfortable speed.

At the beginning of each resting interval, the Borg CR10 scale was asked from the volunteer. Hence, 10 Borg values were obtained at the end of the test. A Zephyr HxM BT (Medtronic, USA) sensor was placed on the subject's chest using an elastic band, for measuring his heart rate during the whole test, by a Bluetooth communication channel with a sampling frequency of 1 Hz. Besides, one Shimmer3 IMU Unit was located on the thigh of the subject's dominant leg (the right one) with an elastic band. The three accelerometers, three gyroscopes, and the EMG module of the Shimmer3 were set to provide their data with a sampling rate of 512 Hz, through a Bluetooth communication channel. Finally, three external electrodes were attached to the corresponding leg, two on the biceps femoris and one to the external protuberance of the femur, as the reference of the EMG signals. The setup of the study can be seen in Figure 6.6.

6.5.3.2 Results of the Anaerobic Study

According to the previous section, five types of metrics were measured. The raw signals of these measurements can be seen in Figure 6.7, where the dashed lines

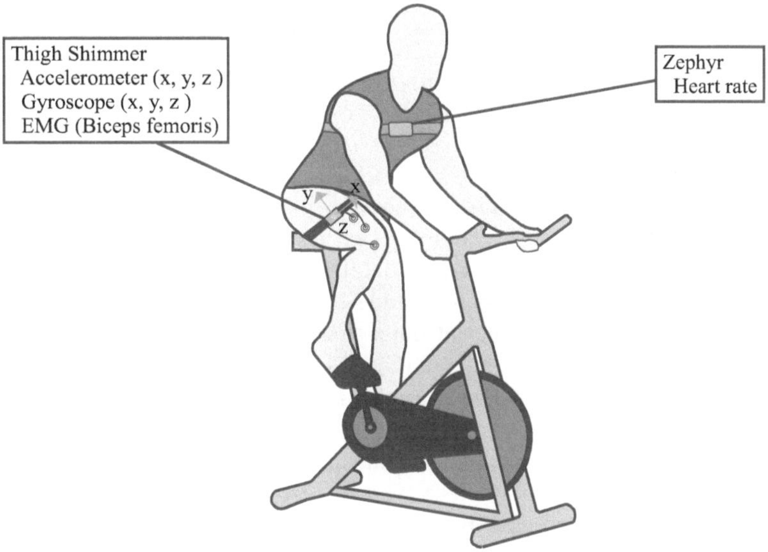

FIGURE 6.6 Anaerobic study setup. Participant was instrumented with an IMU placed on the thigh of his dominant side, and a heart rate sensor located on the middle of the chest.

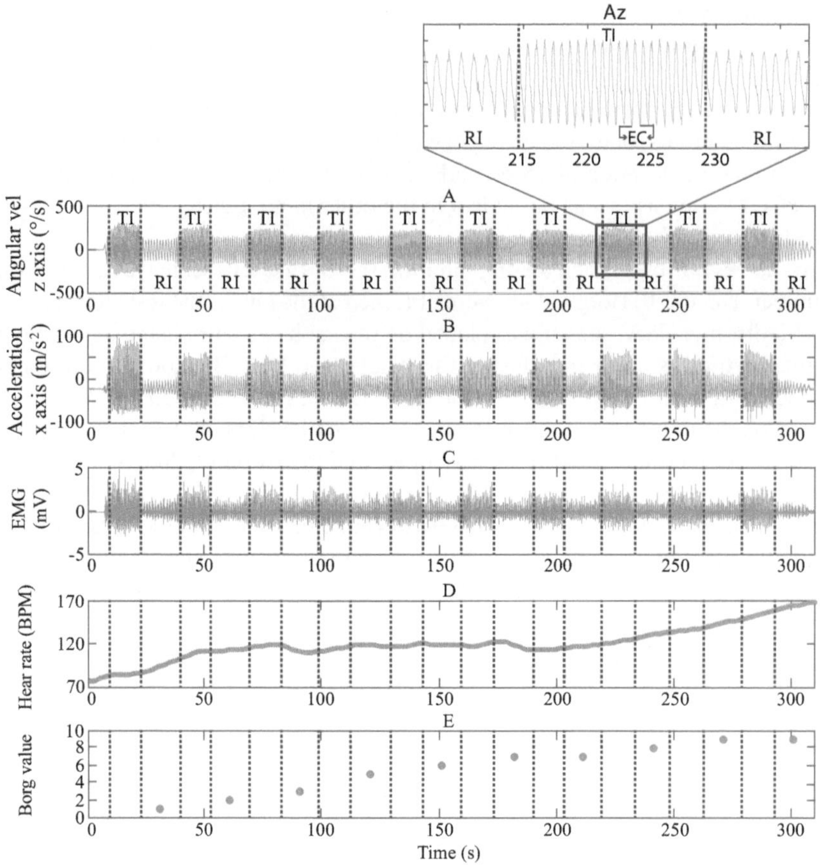

FIGURE 6.7 Anaerobic cycle test signals. (A) gyroscope of the z-axis, (B) accelerometer of the x-axis, (C) electromyography of the right biceps femoris, (D) heart rate and (E) Borg values.

divide the Training Intervals (TIs) and the Resting Intervals (RIs). Plot (A), shows the gyroscope of the z-axis. It was the signal used for determining the beginning and the end of each interval because it contains less noise, and the intervals can be distinguished easily through the amplitude and frequency of the signal. Plot (B) contains the accelerometer signal of the x-axis, which presents a similar shape to the gyroscope with more noise. In plot (C), it is possible to see the right biceps femoris electromyography, which also increases in the training intervals; nevertheless, to get a better interpretation of this signal, a power analysis is required. Plot (D) presents the heart rate of the volunteer during the test. Finally, plot (E) shows the 10 Borg values asked from volunteer every resting interval. It can be appreciated with these two final measurements that the volunteer presented a continued fatigue increment during the test.

In the first place, the fatigue perception (quantified with the Borg CR10 scale) incremented or remained equal regarding the previous resting interval, which means that the volunteer felt exhausted after each training interval. Besides, it is essential to highlight the difference between the first (1 BS value) and the last (9 BS value) Borg scales obtained, showing that the volunteer changed from a low to a high fatigue perceived level in less than 5 minutes, eliciting the anaerobic metabolism.

Similar behavior is shown for the heart rate results (Figure 6.7D), where it is possible to see that the resting heart rate is around 70 BPM at the beginning of the test, and finished near the 170 BPM, which represents approximately the 80% of the heart rate reserve. Furthermore, from the training interval 1 to 3, and from the 7 to 10, the heart rate increased continuously, showing that the volunteer's body required to use more energy for continuing with the test. However, during the other consecutive intervals (4 to 6), it can be appreciated that the heart rate took values close to 120 BPM, which is approximately the 41% of the heart rate reserve, without significant changes. This suggests that during this part of the test, the body was able to create enough energy for executing the activity and the other essential life tasks.

Figure 6.8 presents a percentage of decrease of the following signals: the RMS of the EMG signal, the accelerometer magnitude, and the gyroscope magnitude. In order to get this percentage of decrease, an initial training interval was used to get the initial value of the corresponding signal 6.5; hence, after normalizing the data, the value represented is 0% for this interval. Plot (A) contains the average of the maximum values of each EMG contraction, implementing an RMS mobile window with a size of 100 milliseconds. Therefore, each dot represents the mean power during the training intervals. In plot (B), it is possible to see how the average of the magnitude angular velocity is changing in each training interval, which was estimated for each cycle with the three gyroscopes (x, y, and z) and Equation 6.4. Finally, plot (C) shows the average acceleration magnitude, implementing the same methodology for the angular velocity.

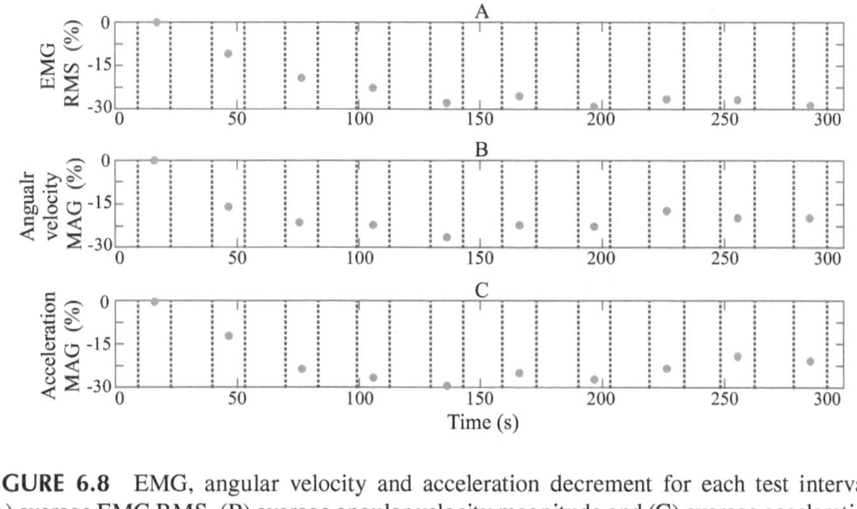

FIGURE 6.8 EMG, angular velocity and acceleration decrement for each test interval, (A) average EMG RMS, (B) average angular velocity magnitude and (C) average acceleration magnitude.

It can be seen in Figure 6.8 how the three average metrics display a similar behavior from the interval 1 to 5, showing continued decrease. Then EMG RMS power analysis remains almost constant, which reflects that the muscle reached a fatigued state. On the other hand, the angular velocity and the acceleration started to increase from the 7th interval, suggesting that the volunteer was able to do the exercise with a better performance. This increment is related to the heart rate behavior because during this part the volunteer could have been forced to change the execution technique of the exercise, in order to incorporate other muscles that help him keep performing the activity, which required him to use more energy, and thus, to increment the heart rate and the fatigue perception.

From this part, it can be considered that the volunteer was over-training and reaching extreme exercise conditions in the context of rehabilitation scenarios, especially because the heart rate signal presented an uncontrolled incremental behavior. However, the volunteer was in the resting intervals. Therefore, the idea would be to stop in those intervals where the signals presented a constant behavior and a secure state (from interval 4 to 6) that can be easily detected with the IMU sensors, owing to, in these sections, the signals presented the lowest values without significant changes.

Thus, this experiment shows the relationship that some IMU performance features have different methods for fatigue estimation during an anaerobic exercise, and how these measurements can be used to detect non-desired fatigued states during the rehabilitation process.

6.6 DISCUSSION

Physical exercise is considered a fundamental part of the different rehabilitation processes in order to improve patients' quality of life. However, the intensity of physical exercise should be regulated. Hence, it is required to implement methods that allow monitoring of rehabilitation therapies because high states of fatigue can harm the patient's rehabilitation and health. Taking into account the context of this problematic, this chapter presented some strategies used to measure fatigue and the most commonly used instruments. With the realization of this work, it was expected to demonstrate the exercise performance strategy using inertial measurement units. The study was made in order to illustrate that muscular fatigue can be measured with the inertial measurement unit, and these results help to improve this field. Also, it is expected that based on these results, these systems will be potentially used in rehabilitation settings to ensure proper monitoring and success in the therapy.

Throughout the development of this chapter, the importance of physical training and the measure of fatigue was discussed. Similarly, in order to evaluate and analyze fatigue, two proposed experiments based on aerobic and anaerobic exercises were described and deployed. Regarding the results presented in the previous section, there are significant findings related to exercise performance.

In both studies, the muscular activity registered a decrease in the activation of electrical activity when the participants started to present fatigue. The maximum decrease in muscular activity was 52% in aerobic results vs. 31% in anaerobic results. Also, when the muscle reached a fatigued state, the muscular activity remained almost constant, as shown in the anaerobic study. According to the results illustrated in the aerobic study, the spatiotemporal parameters such as cadence and the duration of the gait phases (stance and swing) are affected. Accurately, the participant's cadence decreases when they feel exhaustion. Fatigue also generates an increase in gait cycle duration, and consequently, the duration of the gait phases increases proportionally. The participant's fatigue was corroborated with the lactate that provides a direct measurement of the subject's exertion during the study. This physiological parameter increased during the session. This means that the fatigue was progressively increased during the study, and the participant felt exhausted at each stage.

Regarding the anaerobic study results, the angular velocity average and the magnitude acceleration illustrated a decrease until the 5th interval. However, after the 6th interval, these parameters started to increase. This suggests that the participant was in the over-training stage; therefore, the participant changed the technical execution and was able to incorporate other muscles to keep performing the activity. However, this is not recommended because it requires using more energy, which can be reflected in the continuous increase of the heart rate, leading the participant to reach risky physiological conditions (80% of the heart rate reserve) for rehabilitation scenarios.

These findings hold promising potential in terms of monitoring the physical performance exhibited by the participants. Finally, one aspect worth mentioning is that in both studies at the end of the last test, the Borg CR10 scale increased almost to its maximum value. This means that the perception of the participant's effort represented an extreme intensity of the activity.

6.7 CONCLUSIONS

This chapter presented the design and application of a strategy corresponding to exercise performance for fatigue estimation. Two experimental studies based on aerobic and anaerobic exercises were carried out. Each system has a distinctive sensory architecture using inertial measurement. It was conducted to illustrate that muscular fatigue can be measured with these systems. Both systems allowed the acquisition of relevant data from the participants, which were processed in order to analyze the participant's performance during the session.

As initial observations, we found the importance of detecting segments to represent exercise intervals, for example, the walking cycle in the case of aerobic exercise or the interval of the cycling cycle concerning anaerobic exercise. Through these segments, it is possible to find the corresponding fatigue estimation parameters. In the same way, essential results showed how it is possible to detect different fatigue-related parameters as spatiotemporal and kinematic using the inertial measurement unit.

Although the results presented in this chapter are promising, this research is still at an early stage. Thus, the findings of this work will serve as the basis to extend our studies to a larger scale. Therefore, as a future step, we propose to validate these outcomes in a higher number of volunteers and implement an automated system for detecting fatigue. This will allow a more robust statistical analysis, providing meaningful information associated with it.

REFERENCES

[1] Hoda M. Abd-Elfattah, Faten H. Abdelazeim, and Shorouk Elshennawy. Physical and cognitive consequences of fatigue: A review. *Journal of Advanced Research*, 6(3):351–358, 2015.

[2] A. Aguirre, J. Casas, N. Céspedes, M. Múnera, M. Rincon-Roncancio, A. Cuesta-Vargas, and C. A. Cifuentes. Feasibility study: Towards estimation of fatigue level in robot-assisted exercise for cardiac rehabilitation. In *2019 IEEE 16th International Conference on Rehabilitation Robotics (ICORR)*, pages 911–916, 2019.

[3] Barbara E. Ainsworth, William L. Haskell, Arthur S. Leon, David R. Jacobs Jr, Henry J. Montoye, James F. Sallis, and Ralph S. Paffenbarger Jr. Compendium of physical activities: classification of energy costs of human physical activities. *Medicine and Science in Sports and Exercise*, 25(1):71–80, 1993.

[4] Barbara E. Ainsworth, William L. Haskell, Melicia C. Whitt, Melinda L. Irwin, Ann M. Swartz, Scott J. Strath, William L. O. Brien, David R. Bassett, Kathryn H. Schmitz, Patricia O. Emplaincourt, et al. Compendium of physical activities: an update of activity codes and met intensities. *Medicine and Science in Sports and Exercise*, 32(9; SUPP/1):S498–S504, 2000.

[5] Abdullah F. Alghannam, Kostas Tsintzas, Dylan Thompson, James Bilzon, and James A. Betts. Exploring mechanisms of fatigue during repeated exercise and the dose dependent effects of carbohydrate and protein ingestion: study protocol for a randomised controlled trial. *Trials*, 15(1):95, 2014.

[6] John Annett. Subjective rating scales: Science or art? *Ergonomics*, 45(14):966–987, 2002.

[7] A. Appels and P. Mulder. Fatigue and heart disease. The association between 'vital exhaustion' and past, present and future coronary heart disease. *Journal of Psychosomatic Research*, 33(6):727–738, 1989.

[8] Monique Badier, Chantal Guillot, Cédric Danger, Ferdinand Tagliarini, and Yves Jammes. *M-wave hanges after high-and low-frequency electrically induced fatigue in different muscles*, volume 22. Wiley Online Library, 1999.

[9] Michael P. Barnes, Bruce H. Dobkin, and Julien Bogousslavsky. *Recovery after stroke, United Kingdom*: Cambridge University Press, 2005.

[10] Louise Baussard, Marion Carayol, Bertrand Porro, Fanny Baguet, and Florence Cousson-gelie. European Journal of Oncology Nursing Fatigue in cancer patients: Development and validation of a short form of the Multidimensional Fatigue Inventory (MFI-10). *European Journal of Oncology Nursing*, 36(July):62–67, 2018.

[11] Clayton L. Camic, Attila J. Kovacs, Trisha A. VanDusseldorp, Ethan C. Hill, and Evan A. Enquist. Application of the neuromuscular fatigue threshold treadmill test to muscles of the quadriceps and hamstrings. *Journal of Sport and Health Science*, 20(4):1–6, June 2017.

[12] J-M. Casillas, S. Damak, J-C. Chauvet-Gelinier, G. Deley, and P. Ornetti. Fatigue in patients with cardiovascular disease. *Annales de Readaptation et de Medecine Physique: Revue Scientifique de la Societe Francaise de Reeducation Fonctionnelle de Readaptation et de Medecine Physique*, 49(6):309–19, 392–402, 2006.

[13] Mario Cifrek, Vladimir Medved, Stanko Tonković, and Saša Ostojić. Surface EMG based muscle fatigue evaluation in biomechanics. *Clinical Biomechanics*, 24(4):327–340, 2009.

[14] Luis Eduardo Cruz-Martínez, Jaime Tomás Rojas-Valencia, Juan Felipe Correa-Mesa, and Juan Carlos Correa-Morales. Maximum heart rate during exercise: Reliability of the 220-age and Tanaka formulas in healthy young people at a moderate elevation. *Revista Facultad de Medicina*, 62(4):579–585, 2014.

[15] Edith H. Cup, Allan J. Pieterse, Jessica M. ten Broek-Pastoor, Marten Munneke, Baziel G. van Engelen, Henk T. Hendricks, Gert J. van derWilt, and Rob A. Oostendorp. Exercise therapy and other types of physical therapy for patients with neuromuscular diseases: A systematic review. *Archives of Physical Medicine and Rehabilitation*, 88(11):1452–1464, 2007.

[16] N. Céspedes, M. Múnera, C. Gómez, and C. A. Cifuentes. Social human-robot interaction for gait rehabilitation. *IEEE Transactions on Neural Systems and Rehabilitation Engineering*, 28(6):1299–1307, 2020.

[17] Felipe Amorim da Cunha, Paulo de Tarso Veras Farinatti, and Adrian W. Midgley. Methodological and practical application issues in exercise prescription using the heart rate reserve and oxygen uptake reserve methods, *Journal of Science and Medicine in Sport*, 14(1):46–57, 2011.

[18] Mary Ann Dalzell, N. Smirnow, W. Sateren, A. Sintharaphone, M. Ibrahim, L. Mastroianni, L. D. Vales Zambrano, and S. O'Brien. Rehabilitation and exercise oncology program: Translating research into a model of care. *Current Oncology*, 24(3):e191–e198, 2017.

[19] Grace Olivia Dibben, Hasnain M. Dalal, Rod S. Taylor, Patrick Doherty, Lars Hermann Tang, and Melvyn Hillsdon. Cardiac rehabilitation and physical activity: Systematic review and meta-analysis, *Heart*, 104(17), 1394–1402, 2018.

[20] W. Dörr, R. Engenhart-Cabillic, and J. S. Zimmermann. Radiotherapy-related fatigue and exercise for cancer patients: a review of the literature and suggestions for future research. *Normal Tissue Reactions in Radiotherapy and Oncology*, 37:49, 2002.

[21] Yaoshan Dun, Joshua R. Smith, Suixin Liu, and Thomas P. Olson. High-intensity interval training in cardiac rehabilitation, *Clinics in Geriatric Medicine*, 35(4): 469–487, 2019.

[22] Yolanda Escalante, Jose M. Saavedra, Antonio García-Hermoso, Antonio J. Silva, and Tiago M. Barbosa. Physical exercise and reduction of pain in adults with lower limb osteoarthritis: A systematic review, *Journal of Back and Musculoskelatal Rehabilitation*, 23(4): 175–186, 2010.

[23] Walter R. Frontera and Howard K. Knuttgen. Exercise and musculoskeletal rehabilitation: Restoring optimal form and function, published online, 2003, doi.org/10.1080/00913847.2003.11439980

[24] Juan García-López, Juan C. Morante, Ana Ogueta-Alday, and Jose A. Rodríguez-Marroyo. The type of mat (contact vs. photocell) affects vertical jump height estimated from flight time. *Journal of Strength and Conditioning Research*, 27(4):1162–1167, 2013.

[25] Asok Kumar Ghosh. Anaerobic threshold: its concept and role in endurance sport. *The Malaysian journal of medical sciences*, 11(1):24–36, 2004.

[26] Rainer Gloeckl, Tessa Schneeberger, Inga Jarosch, and Klaus Kenn. Pulmonary rehabilitation and exercise training in chronic obstructive pulmonary disease, *Deutsches Arzteblatt International*, 115(8): 117–123, 2018.

[27] Matthew L. Goodwin, James E. Harris, Andrés Hernández, and L. Bruce Gladden. Blood lactate measurements and analysis during exercise: A guide for clinicians. *Journal of Diabetes Science and Technology*, 1(4):558–569, 2007.

[28] Thibaut Guiraud, Anil Nigam, Vincent Gremeaux, Philippe Meyer, Martin Juneau, and Laurent Bosquet. High-intensity interval training in cardiac rehabilitation. *Sports medicine*, 42(7):587–605, 2012.

[29] Brian Hanley and Anna K. Mohan. Changes in gait during constant pace treadmill running. *Journal of Strength and Conditioning Research*, 28(5):1219–1225, 2014.

[30] William L. Haskell, I-Min Lee, Russell R. Pate, Kenneth E. Powell, Steven N. Blair, Barry A. Franklin, Caroline A. Macera, Gregory W. Heath, Paul D. Thompson, and Adrian Bauman. Physical activity and public health: updated recommendation for adults from the American College of Sports Medicine and the American Heart Association. *Circulation*, 116(9):1081, 2007.

[31] Jorunn L. Helbostad, Daina L. Sturnieks, Jasmine Menant, Kim Delbaere, Stephen R. Lord, and Mirjam Pijnappels. Consequences of lower extremity and trunk muscle fatigue on balance and functional tasks in older people: A systematic literature review. *BMC Geriatrics*, 10(1):56, 2010.

[32] Louis J. Ignarro, Maria Luisa Balestrieri, and Claudio Napoli. Nutrition, physical activity, and cardiovascular disease: An update, *Cardiovascular Research*, 73(2), 326–340, 2007.

[33] Hideaki Ishii and Yusuke Nishida. Effect of lactate accumulation during exercise induced muscle fatigue on the sensorimotor cortex. *Journal of Physical Therapy Science*, 25(12):1637–1642, 2013.

[34] John M. Jakicic and Amy D. Otto. Physical activity considerations for the treatment and prevention of obesity. *The American Journal of Clinical Nutrition*, 82(1):226S–229S, 2005.

[35] M. Jetté, K. Sidney, and G. Blümchen. Metabolic equivalents (METS) in exercise testing, exercise prescription, and evaluation of functional capacity. *Clinical Cardiology*, 13(8):555–565, 1990.

[36] Seung Rok Kang, Jin-Young Min, Changho Yu, and Tae-Kyu Kwon. Effect of whole body vibration on lactate level recovery and heart rate recovery in rest after intense exercise. *Technology and Health Care*, 25:115–123, July 2017.

[37] J. B. Kostis, A. E. Moreyra, M. T. Amendo, J. Di Pietro, N. Cosgrove, and P. T. Kuo. The effect of age on heart rate in subjects free of heart disease. Studies by ambulatory electrocardiography and maximal exercise stress test. *Circulation*, 65(1):141–145, 1982.

[38] Yun-sang Lee and Seung-won Ahn. The effects of kinesio taping and neuromuscular rehabilitation exercise for patients with acute whiplash-associated disorder. *The Journal of Korean Academy of Orthopedic Manual Physical Therapy*, 22(2):41–49, 2016.

[39] Heather S. Longpré, Jim R. Potvin, and Monica R. Maly. Biomechanical changes at the knee after lower limb fatigue in healthy young women. *Clinical Biomechanics*, 28(4):441–447, 2013.

[40] M.D. Sánchez Manchola, M.J. Pinto Bernal, M. Munera, and C.A. Cifuentes. Gait phase detection for lower-limb exoskeletons using foot motion data from a single inertial measurement unit in hemiparetic individuals. *Sensors*, 19(13):2988, 2019.

[41] Audrey F. Manley. *Physical activity and health: a report of the surgeon general*. Diane Publishing, 1996.

[42] Andrea Mannini and Angelo Maria Sabatini. Gait phase detection and discrimination between walking–jogging activities using hidden Markov models applied to foot motion data from a gyroscope. *Gait & Posture*, 36(4):657–661, 2012.

[43] Ryan S. McGinnis, Stephen M. Cain, Steven P. Davidson, Rachel V. Vitali, Noel C. Perkins, and Scott G. McLean. Quantifying the effects of load carriage and fatigue under load on sacral kinematics during countermovement vertical jump with IMU-based method. *Sports Engineering*, 19(1):21–34, 2016.

[44] Mark Melnyk and Albert Gollhofer. Submaximal fatigue of the hamstrings impairs specific reflex components and knee stability. *Knee Surgery, Sports Traumatology, Arthroscopy*, 15(5):525–532, 2007.

[45] Felix Möhler, Steffen Ringhof, Daniel Debertin, and Thorsten Stein. Influence of fatigue on running coordination: A UCM analysis with a geometric 2D model and a subject specific anthropometric 3D model. *Human movement science*, 66:133–141, 2019.

[46] Gary R. Morrow, Abhay R. Shelke, Joseph A. Roscoe, Jane T. Hickok, and Karen Mustian. Management of cancer-related fatigue, *Cancer Investigation*, 23(3), 229–239, 2005.

[47] Alvaro Muro-de-la Herran, Begonya Garcia-Zapirain, and Amaia Mendez-Zorrilla. Gait analysis methods: An overview of wearable and non-wearable systems, highlighting clinical applications. *Sensors*, 14(2):3362–3394, 2014.

[48] Richard Nelesen, Yasmin Dar, KaMala Thomas, and Joel E. Dimsdale. The relationship between fatigue and cardiac functioning. *Archives of Internal Medicine*, 168(9):943, 2008.

[49] American College of Sports Medicine et al. *ACSM's health-related physical fitness assessment manual*. Lippincott Williams & Wilkins, 2013.

[50] Ozge Ozalp, Deniz Inal-Ince, Ebru Calik, Naciye Vardar-Yagli, Melda Saglam, Sema Savci, Hulya Arikan, Meral Bosnak-Guclu, and Lutfi Coplu. Extrapulmonary features of bronchiectasis: muscle function, exercise capacity, fatigue, and health status. *Multidisciplinary respiratory medicine*, 7(1):3, 2012.

[51] Bente K. Pedersen. Physical exercise in chronic diseases. In *Nutrition and Skeletal Muscle*, pages 217–266. Elsevier, Jan 2019.

[52] S. Pettersson, I. E. Lundberg, M. H. Liang, J. Pouchot, and E. Welin Henriksson. Determination of the minimal clinically important difference for seven measures of fatigue in Swedish patients with systemic lupus erythematosus. *Scandinavian Journal of Rheumatology*, 44(3):206–210, 2015.

[53] Michael L. Pollock, Glenn A. Gaesser, Janus D. Butcher, Jean Pierre Després, Rod K. Dishman, Barry A. Franklin, and Carol Ewing Garber. The recommended quantity and quality of exercise for developing and maintaining cardiorespiratory and muscular fitness, and flexibility in healthy adults, *Medicine and Science in Sports and Exercise*, 30(6), 975–991,1998.

[54] Kym Joanne Price, Brett Ashley Gordon, Stephen Richard Bird, and Amanda Clare Benson. A review of guidelines for cardiac rehabilitation exercise programmes: Is there an international consensus?, *European Journal of Preventive Cardiology*, 23(16), 1715–1733, 2016.

[55] Xingda Qu and Joo Chuan Yeo. Effects of load carriage and fatigue on gait characteristics. *Journal of Biomechanics*, 44(7):1259–1263, 2011.

[56] Mamun Bin Ibne Reaz, M. Sazzad Hussain, and Faisal Mohd-Yasin. Techniques of EMG signal analysis: detection, processing, classification and applications. *Biological Procedures Online*, 8(1):11–35, 2006.

[57] T. Reybrouck, L. Mertens, S. Brusselle, M. Weymans, B. Eyskens, J. Defoor, and M. Gewillig. Oxygen uptake versus exercise intensity: A new concept in assessing cardiovascular exercise function in patients with congenital heart disease. *Heart*, 84(1):46–52, 2000.

[58] Ganesh Roy, Aritra Bhuiya, Aditya Mukherjee, and Subhasis Bhaumik. Kinect camera based gait data recording and analysis for assistive robotics-an alternative to goniometer based measurement technique. *Procedia Computer Science*, 133:763–771, 2018.

[59] Didier Saey, Annie Michaud, Annabelle Couillard, Claude H. Côté, M. Jeffery Mador, Pierre LeBlanc, Jean Jobin, and François Maltais. Contractile fatigue, muscle morphometry, and blood lactate in chronic obstructive pulmonary disease. *American Journal of Respiratory and Critical Care Medicine*, 171(10):1109–1115, 2005.

[60] Patrick D. Savage, Michael J. Toth, and Philip A. Ades. A re-examination of the metabolic equivalent concept in individuals with coronary heart disease. *Journal of Cardiopulmonary Rehabilitation and Prevention*, 27(3):143–148, 2007.

[61] Yves Schutz, Roland L. Weinsier, and Gary R. Hunter. Assessment of free-living physical activity in humans: An overview of currently available and proposed new measures, *Obesity*, 9(6), 368–379, 2001.

[62] Aida Sehle, Manfred Vieten, Simon Sailer, Annegret Mündermann, and Christian Dettmers. Objective assessment of motor fatigue in multiple sclerosis: the Fatigue index Kliniken Schmieder (FKS). *Journal of Neurology*, 261(9):1752–1762, 2014.

[63] Alsayed A. Shanb and Enas F. Youssef. The impact of adding weight-bearing exercise versus nonweight bearing programs to the medical treatment of elderly patients with osteoporosis. *Journal of Family and Community Medicine*, 21(3):176, 2014.

[64] E. M.A. Smets, B. Garssen, B. Bonke, and J. C.J.M. De Haes. The Multidimensional Fatigue Inventory (MFI) psychometric qualities of an instrument to assess fatigue. *Journal of Psychosomatic Research*, 39(3):315–325, 1995.

[65] Rosalind R. Spence, Kristiann C. Heesch, and Wendy J. Brown. Exercise and cancer rehabilitation: A systematic review. *Cancer Treatment Reviews*, 36(2):185–194, 2010.

[66] Martijn A. Spruit, Fabio Pitta, Edward McAuley, Richard L. ZuWallack, and Linda Nici. Pulmonary rehabilitation and physical activity in patients with chronic obstructive pulmonary disease. *American Thoracic Society*, 192(8):924–933, 2015.

[67] Paul D. Thompson, David Buchner, Ileana L. Pina, Gary J. Balady, Mark A. Williams, Bess H. Marcus, Kathy Berra, Steven N. Blair, Fernando Costa, Barry Franklin, Gerald F. Fletcher, Neil F. Gordon, Russell R. Pate, Beatriz L. Rodriguez, Antronette K. Yancey, and Nanette K. Wenger. Exercise and physical activity in the prevention and treatment of atherosclerotic cardiovascular disease. *Circulation*, 107(24):3109–3116, 2003.

[68] Eric L. Voorn, Fieke Koopman, Frans Nollet, and Merel A. Brehm. Aerobic exercise in adult neuromuscular rehabilitation: A survey of healthcare professionals. *Journal of Rehabilitation Medicine*, 51(7):518–524, 2019.

[69] Jing-jing Wan, Zhen Qin, Peng-yuan Wang, Yang Sun, and Xia Liu. Muscle fatigue: general understanding and treatment. *Experimental & Molecular Medicine*, 49(10):e384–e384, 2017.

[70] Darren E. R. Warburton, Crystal Whitney Nicol, and Shannon S. D. Bredin. Prescribing exercise as preventive therapy. *CMAJ*, 174(7):961–974, 2006.

[71] Darren E. R. Warburton, Norman Gledhill, and Arthur Quinney. Musculoskeletal fitness and health. *Canadian Journal of Applied Physiology*, 26(2):217–237, 2001.

[72] Darren E. R. Warburton, Norman Gledhill, and Arthur Quinney. The effects of changes in musculoskeletal fitness on health. *Canadian Journal of Applied Physiology*, 26(2):161–216, 2001.

[73] Darren E. R. Warburton, Donald C. McKenzie, Mark J. Haykowsky, Arlana Taylor, Paula Shoemaker, Andrew P. Ignaszewski, and Sammy Y. Chan. Effectiveness of high intensity interval training for the rehabilitation of patients with coronary artery disease. *American Journal of Cardiology*, 95(9):1080–1084, 2005.

[74] Nerys Williams. The Borg rating of perceived exertion (RPE) scale. *Occupational Medicine*, 67(5):404–405, 2017.

[75] Sara C. Winter, James B. Lee, Raymond I. Leadbetter, and Susan J. Gordon. Validation of a single inertial sensor for measuring running kinematics overground during a prolonged run, 5(1): 1423, 2016.

[76] Petra Wirtz and Freerk T. Baumann. Physical activity, exercise and breast cancer - what is the evidence for rehabilitation, aftercare, and survival? A review. *Breast Care*, 13(2):93–101, 2018.

[77] Edward M. Wojtys, Bradford B. Wylie, and Laura J. Huston. The effects of muscle fatigue on neuromuscular function and anterior tibial translation in healthy knees. *The American Journal of Sports Medicine*, 24(5):615–621, 1996.

[78] World Health Organization. Physical activity, 2016 (accessed February 25, 2016). https://www.who.int/news-room/fact-sheets/detail/physical-activity.

[79] Fei Yu, Arne Bilberg, Egon Stenager, Chiara Rabotti, Bin Zhang, and Massimo Mischi. A wireless body measurement system to study fatigue in multiple sclerosis. *Physiological Measurement*, 33(12):2033–2048, 2012.

[80] Antonio Roberto Zamunér, Marlene Aparecida Moreno, Taís M. Camargo, Juliana Paula Graetz, Ana Cristina Silva Rebelo, Nayara Yamada Tamburús, and Ester da Silva. Assessment of subjective perceived exertion at the anaerobic threshold with the Borg CR-10 scale. *Journal of Sports Science Medicine*, 10(1):130–136, 2011.

7 Conversational Agents for Healthcare Delivery: Potential Solutions to the Challenges of the Pandemic

Margarita Bautista[1], Carlos A. Cifuentes[1], and Marcela Munera[1]

[1]Department of Biomedical Engineering, Colombian School of Engineering Julio Garavito, Bogotá, Colombia.

CONTENTS

7.1 Introduction 112
7.2 Methods 114
7.2.1 Sources and Searching 115
7.2.2 Inclusion and Exclusion Criteria 115
7.2.3 Assessment of Review Quality 116
7.2.4 Data Extraction 116
7.3 Classification of Conversational Agents for Healthcare 116
7.3.1 Education and Counseling 120
7.3.2 Rehabilitation 123
7.3.3 Mental Health 126
7.3.4 Physical Training 126
7.3.5 Palliative Care 128
7.4 Future Works 129
7.4.1 Limitations 129
7.4.2 Recommendations 130
7.5 Conclusions 130
References 131

7.1 INTRODUCTION

In the 1950s, research in Artificial Intelligence (AI) was supported by a group of scientists and researchers who predicted that machines would be capable, in just a few decades, of carrying out any task that humans could. Nevertheless, it was not until 60 years later that the trend of Conversational Agents (CAs) started with Siri (Apple, 2011) [51], which provided a speech interface for question answering. Following Apple, some companies, including Google, AT&T, Nuance, among others, have successfully participated in the market of smart CAs [25] creating awareness in millions of consumers that indeed smartphones could speak, answer limited set of questions, execute simple tasks and, in some cases, be friendly.

Since the creation of the first CAs, their common functionality was their capacity to interpret natural language via spoken interaction and to provide responses either in the form of running a software program (e.g., making calls, sending text messages, setting reminders, etc.) or a spoken response (question answering like, "*What is the capital of Colombia?*", or "*Which is the nearest Colombian restaurant?*") [25]. Over time, interest in offering better services increased, and in response, the idea of personifying CAs was revolutionary [14] giving rise to the Embodied Conversational Agents (ECAs).

An example of an early ECA is SimCoach (USC Institute for Creative Technologies, 2013) [22], which was created in response to healthcare challenges generated by the conflicts in Iraq and Afghanistan in the U.S. population. The SimCoach project developed different archetypes of support agents to serve as online guides for assisting the military and their families to initiate the healthcare process [53]. Despite its potential use, it was not conceived to deliver diagnosis or treatment, or as a replacement for human providers and experts.

Currently, ECAs are not the only name given to CAs, according to their technical characteristics they can also be called *chatbot* [32], *avatar* [64], *virtual human* [29], among others [25]. Despite the different names they may receive, the definitions are rather similar using variations of character that demonstrates many of the same properties as humans in a face-to-face conversation. The most relevant characteristic similar to humans is their ability to produce and respond to verbal and non-verbal communication.

As CAs evolved, so did wearable devices; advances such as heart rate monitors, smartwatches, activity monitors, and other wearable sensors, have made mobile devices ideal units for healthcare delivery [48, 51]; this and working together with CAs open up a new and growing world of possibilities. For example, there are currently a large number of applications that can track user activity, eating habits and analyze signals such as blood pressure, heart rate, respiratory rate, skin temperature, etc., by interacting with various wearable devices as shown in Figure 7.1.

The use of wearable devices has been emerging rapidly due to their potential to improve the level of healthcare delivery and reducing costs. For this reason, the possibility of innovation by means of using wearable devices with the intervention of CAs could allow in some cases immediate feedback, supplementing the shortage of staff in primary healthcare centers and thereby reducing the burden on service providers.

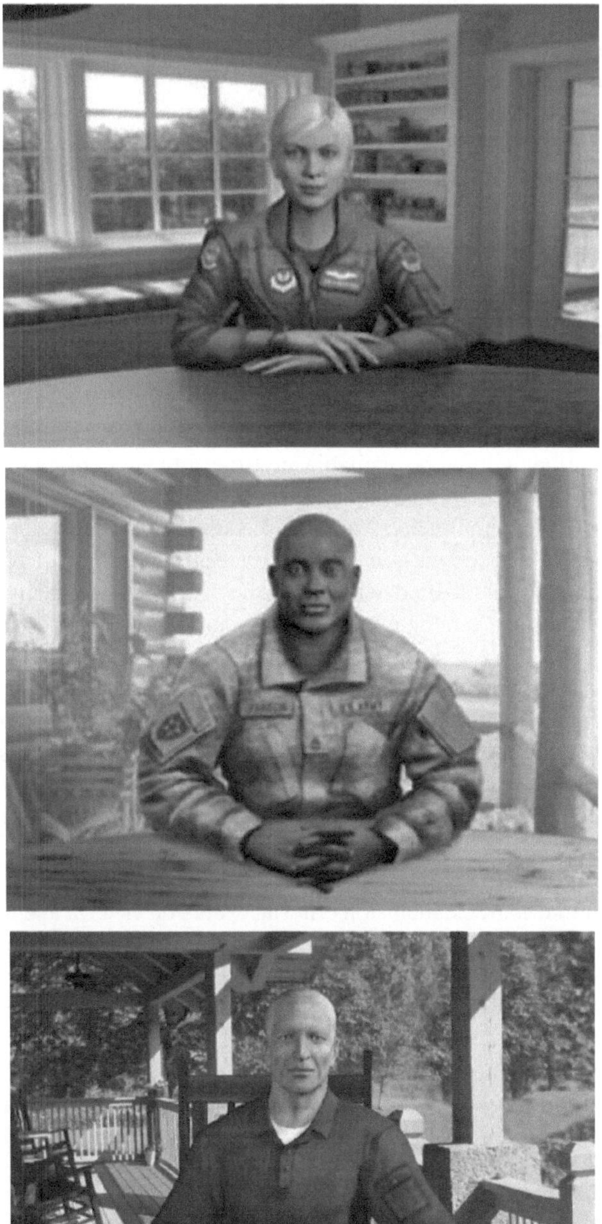

FIGURE 7.1 Common architecture for the integration of wearable sensors and mobile devices for healthcare monitoring.

Considering the current situation, the COVID-19 pandemic is considered as the most crucial global health calamity of the century and the greatest challenge that humankind has faced since the Second World War [15]. According to the report of the World Health Organization (WHO), the current outbreak of COVID-19 has affected over 2,164,111 people and killed more than 146,198 people in more than 200 countries throughout the world [46]. Almost all nations are struggling to stop the transmission of the disease through testing, treatment of patients and social isolation [15]. These preventive measures have generated enormous health, economic and social challenges for the entire human population. Accordingly, at this point in time, it is indispensable to develop alternatives as mentioned in the previous paragraph to resume essential activities such as those in the area of health geared towards monitoring of chronic patients or rehabilitation processes.

What makes this new way of healthcare delivery ideal for supporting people in some processes is its capacity of establishing and maintaining an empathic relationship [30]. In addition, it could be available anytime, anywhere offering support when it matters most which maximizes impact [51]. However, despite the promising role it can play in supporting people, literature that discusses how to develop it and demonstrates its long-term effectiveness is scarce [30]. Although in most of the literature, users report being fully satisfied with CAs, they do not necessarily translate into improvements in clinical outcome (e.g., a significant reduction in a clinical measure of depression).

This chapter is organized in five sections, addressing a systematic review of the different medical applications in which the integration of wearable devices and CAs creates a new way to healthcare delivery through interactive and personalized support that can be carried out in both hospital and home conditions. Also, it provides an overview of their efficacy and use-related outcomes in early experiments or pilot studies.

Section 7.2 presents the methodology used to conduct the systematic review considering aspects like sources, inclusion criteria, exclusion criteria and data extraction.

Section 7.3 presents a review of studies related to CAs for medical applications paying particular attention to systems that integrate wearable devices, their classification according to the domain area and some practical characteristics.

Section 7.4 discusses some recommendations for future works that were identified based on the results of this review.

Finally, Section 7.5 presents the conclusions reached and the challenges of the use of wearable devices in joint work with CAs.

7.2 METHODS

The systematic review is focused on CAs that may or may not work in conjunction with wearable devices for medical applications, given their growing availability and use. Based on the literature, there is no consensus on the definitions of CAs; as a consequence, different names are used to call them. According to their technical characteristics, some examples of names are: embodied conversational agent, animated character, virtual avatar, and chatbot, among others. That is why, in order to collect as much information as possible, all types of CAs will be included, regardless of the type of communication (verbal, non-verbal, written and visual), as long as the purpose is geared towards the health sector.

Although there is no consensus in the literature on definitions of CAs, there is an agreement in the literature on the methodology to be followed. Based on the above, an adequate systematic review of scientific papers should consider the following aspects: sources and searching, inclusion and exclusion criteria, assessment of review quality, and data extraction [58].

7.2.1 Sources and Searching

An electronic search was conducted in April 2020 using Scopus, Science Direct, IEEE, ACM Digital and PubMed databases about CAs for healthcare delivery. Search terms included conversational agent, virtual agent, virtual human, virtual therapist, virtual coaching, dialogue system, relational agent, chatbot and their combinations with the word healthcare. Similarly, the reference lists of relevant articles were taken into account to be searched. In addition, wildcard symbols, such as hyphens or inverted commas, were used to consider all possible variations of root words.

The key terms used for the literature search are clearly described below:

(*"conversational agent*"* **OR** *"virtual agent*"* **OR** *"virtual human*"* **OR** *"virtual therapist*"* **OR** *"virtual coaching*"* **OR** *"dialogue system*"* **OR** *"relational agent*"* **OR** *chatbot**) **AND** *"healthcare*"*

7.2.2 Inclusion and Exclusion Criteria

The review focuses on all type of CAs that use natural or non-natural language input, without any restrictions, given their increasing availability and use by consumers, caregivers or healthcare professionals. Some examples of the types of CAs that are considered are (but are not limited to): chatbots, which have the ability to engage in a short and casual conversation; embodied conversational agents, which involve a computer-generated character (e.g., avatar, virtual agent) simulating face-to-face conversation with verbal and non-verbal communication; and smart conversational interfaces such as Apple's Siri, Google Now, Microsoft Cortana, or Amazon Alexa.

According to the foregoing, articles obtained through these searches were evaluated using the title and abstract. The articles were included in this systematic review when they met the following criteria:

The study must be focused on CAs for healthcare delivery.

The study must include at least an experiment, a pilot study or a trial with at least one group of participants.

The study must present the methodology and report the results of quantitative or qualitative assessments of human user interaction with the CA.

It should be noted that there is no restriction on year of publication or language.

TABLE 7.1
Criteria for Methodological Evaluation

Criteria	Possible Outcomes		
Was there a clear statement of the aims of the research?	1	0.5	0
Is a qualitative methodology appropriate?	1	0.5	0
Is the sample/population identified and appropriate?	1	0.5	0
Is there a clear statement of findings?	1	0.5	0
Are the results accurate?	1	0.5	0

Note: 1 stands for *Yes*, 0 stands for *No* and 0.5 stands for *Not Applicable* or *Cannot Tell*

7.2.3 Assessment of Review Quality

The quality and scope of all studied documents varies widely. Nevertheless, when assessing the quality of the reviews, efforts should be made to avoid the influence of external variables such as authors, institutional affiliations, and journal names, among others.

Given the nature of this review, the existing literature suggests a quality assessment called Critical Appraisal Skills Programme (CASP) Systematic Review Checklist [1], which is ideal to assess the quality of the included documents to help ensure the strength of the evidence. In particular, studied publications were subject to five criteria, as shown in Table 7.1.

7.2.4 Data Extraction

Firstly, an initial review of the articles was conducted based on the information contained in their titles and abstracts. Subsequently, a full reading of the text was performed to identify which studies were included or excluded according to the criteria set out above. Additionally, to ensure the strength of the evidence, the documents included were assessed using the CASP checklist. Finally, the following data were extracted from the documents that were included in the review: first author, year of publication, domain area, target population, type of conversation agent, methodology, duration of the study, measures of evaluation and conclusion. With the information extracted, the document began to be written, separating studies according to the scenario for which they were used, and highlighting those studies that involved wearable devices.

7.3 CLASSIFICATION OF CONVERSATIONAL AGENTS FOR HEALTHCARE

Recent advancements in natural language recognition and synthesis have resulted in the adoption of CAs in different areas of our daily life, such as in science, commerce, and service, among others [51]. Added to this, the rising popularity of these technologies has been facilitated by a renaissance in AI [37], the development of powerful processors supporting deep learning algorithms, and technological advancements that make a wealth of computational knowledge available within reach.

Currently, one emerging area where CAs have potential to help address some shortages and unmet needs is in the health sector, especially in healthcare services delivery because of their abilities to (i) imitate conversation with humans through natural language, (ii) be available any time, anywhere and (iii) provide an almost immediate response [26]. This field is still in a nascent period of investigation, that is why most studied documents have been publised after 2005 and rarely evaluate efficacy or safety. Nonetheless, CAs have been widely used with success in industy for dissemination of news, offers and promotions, and in the commerce for customer service [31, 51].

Despite the fact that the literature of CAs for healthcare services delivery is scarce, most of the research in this area is on education and counseling, which are used to support patients and clinicians in highly specific processes. Moreover, some other research evaluates CAs for rehabilitation, mental health, physical training and palliative care, ordered according to the amount of information found. Overall, the published studies suggest that CAs can make an intervention more engaging, although evidence on their effectiveness remains inconclusive. In the same way, all studies have measured user experience by linking the level of acceptance and comfort with the participation of CAs. In some studies, the Likert Scale was the methodology used to measure people's opinions and attitudes [54]. In some other cases, Acceptability E-Scale (AES) was used for assessing the level of acceptability of the CAs from patients [49]. However, regardless of the scale used, participants expressed comfort in interacting with CAs and were very receptive to them [57].

Although there is a good user perception of CAs, their potential largely depends on whether these technologies are accessible to the populations that could benefit from them. Therefore, in most cases, CAs rely on different types of technology including Apps delivered via mobile device [9], web [53], or computer [16, 21], Short Message Service (SMS) [50] and telephone [7]. As shown in Figure 7.2, of the technologies mentioned above, two are ideal for healthcare delivery due to their easy access and global character. The first technology is web-based, which is the best if you want to reach as many people and devices as possible with minimum hassle [36]. The second one is mobile devices which represent a great alternative because they are omnipresent and the user can be reached by the CAs at all times and in all places [10], both with the limitation that in most cases an Internet connection is needed.

Just as there are different types of technologies that support virtual agents, the authors of the studies found also use of different names to refer to CAs; examples of this include *embodied conversational agent* [7, 9, 11, 12, 34, 59, 65], *virtual human* [29, 35, 49, 52, 53, 60, 66], *animated character* [24, 57, 62, 63], *virtual avatar* [17, 20, 64], *virtual agent* [18, 33, 61], *automated conversational agent* [21, 56], *natural dialogue system* [13, 50], *artificial conversational agent* [27], *relational agent* [8], and *chatbot* [16], among others [19, 55]. But the purpose of these is the same: create a new way of health service delivery by supporting patients and clinicians in some activities without substituting their role.

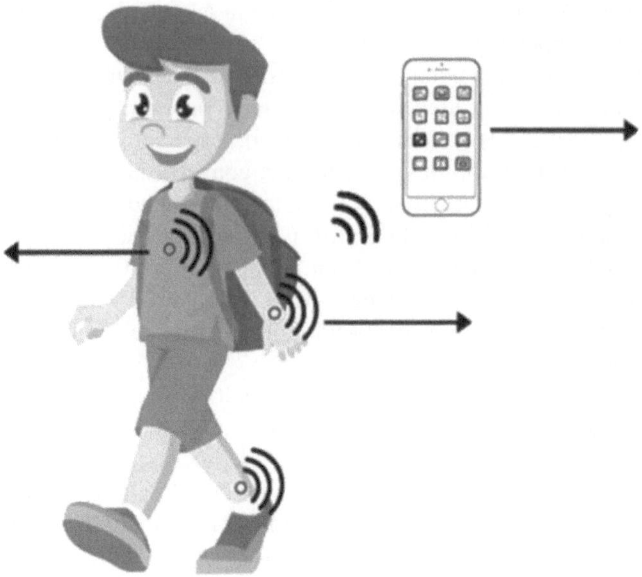

FIGURE 7.2 Conversation agents delivered by different platforms depending on the purpose of the agent and the activity to be performed. a) Conversational Agent delivered via mobile device to provide attention, advice and motivation anytime, anywhere. b) Conversational Agent delivered via web to exemplify activities aimed at physical exercise and rehabilitation at any time.

Regarding the integration of wearable devices with CAs, few studies are found in the literature, only two recent studies clearly show an integrated system between wearable devices and CAs. Both studies were proposed in 2018 by Shamekhi et al. [56] and Bickmore et al. [9]. Firstly, Shamekhi et al. presented a CA that acts as a virtual meditation coach for alleviating symptoms related to a variety of chronic health conditions, including pain, anxiety, and depression. Based on study, meditation takes practice and requires regular training that most people cannot perform. For these reasons, the designed CA can be used at any time, if a computer is available. Additionaly, the CA is interactive and adaptive to a user's breathing behavior, based on inputs from a respiration sensor as shown in Figure 7.3.

The respiration sensor is used to calculate the user's breathing rate so that the coach can provide feedback on it at key points during the meditation. As a result of this study, participants felt that the virtual meditation coach was significantly more aware of their status when it incorporated information from a respiration sensor in its customized training. In the same way, participants also reported that their meditation was significantly more relaxing and helpful when the coach responded to their breathing. Regarding the level of acceptance, to evaluate the users' reactions to the virtual meditation instructor, a questionnaire was conducted from 1 (not at all satisfied) to 7 (very satisfied), scoring it with an average of 6.11. In view of the above, these results indicate that users were highly receptive to the CA and appreciated the interactivity afforded by the respiration sensor.

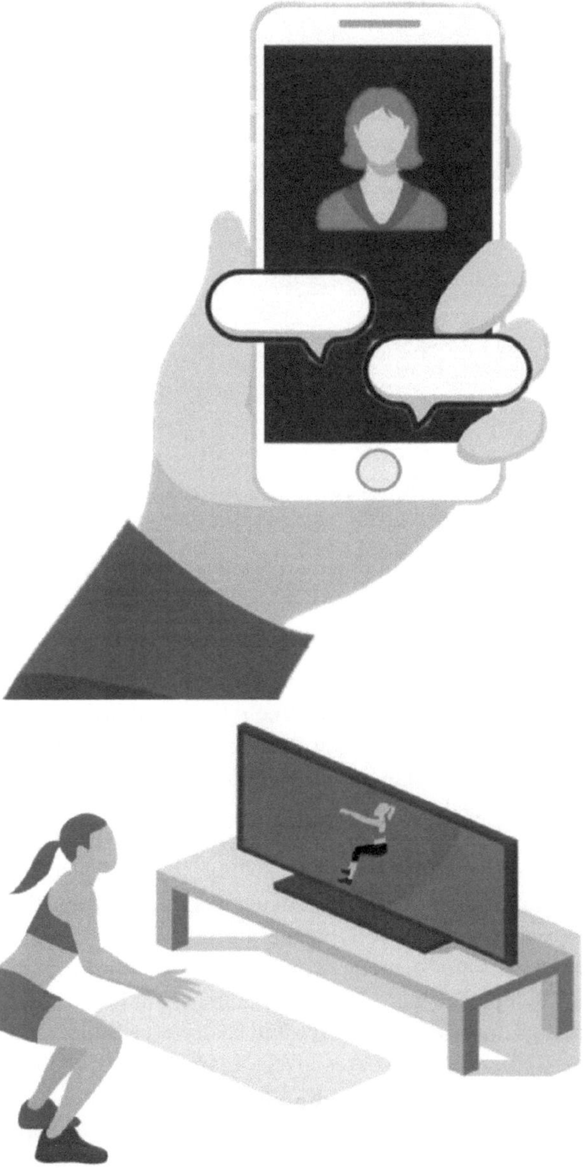

FIGURE 7.3 Experimental setup proposed by Shamekhi et al. for guide meditation sessions based on the input from respiration sensor.

Later, Bickmore et al. proposed a system that integrated a CA and a heart rhythm monitor called Kardia (AliveCor, 2017) [3] to advise patients with Atrial Fibrillation (AF) on self-management of their disease. According to experts, the correct management of this chronic condition is essential to prevent strokes, heart failure and sudden death. That is why this system is an excellent alternative to allow individuals to

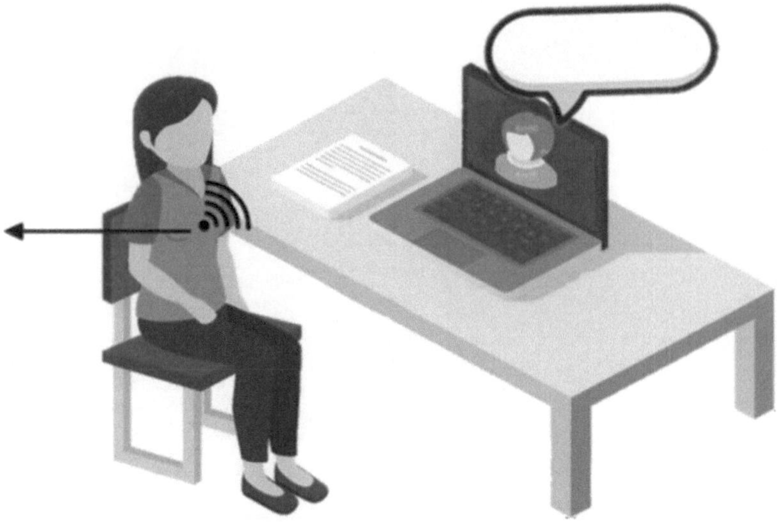

FIGURE 7.4 Experimental setup proposed by Bickmore et al. for advising patients with atrial fibrillation based on the input from a heart rhythm monitor.

better manage their condition through: (i) frequent monitoring of heart rhythm and (ii) the dialogue about important topics like AF education, symptom report, medications intake and potential emergencies that may arise. As shown in Figure 7.4, the designed system can be used at anytime and anywhere from a cell phone, assisting the user whenever needed.

Based on results of this study, participants regularly used the system, reported symptoms continuously, and were very satisfied. Regarding to the satisfaction level with the agent, a questionnaire was conducted from 1 (very unsatisfied) to 7 (very satisfied), rating it with a median of 5. Furthermore, to understand how the participants felt about the CA, an interview was conducted in which the participants expressed their opinions. Most participants reported that the agent was friendly and appropriate, therapeutic and comforting, informative and easily accessible, among others.

Considering that chronic diseases affect a large part of the population, and programs for the self-management of these diseases are complex, CAs and wearable devices are important tools that used together can improve population health and decrease healthcare costs.

A summary of other studies which do not integrate wearable devices is featured below, showing an overview of CAs and their progress over the years in certain health domains.

7.3.1 Education and Counseling

According to the WHO, 41 million people die each year from non-communicable diseases such as cardiovascular disease, cancer, chronic respiratory disease and diabetes [43]. That death toll corresponds to 71% of all deaths globally, a worrying figure given that in most cases these deaths could be avoided with self-care education and counseling.

These diseases are the result of a combination of genetic, physiological, environmental and behavioral factors that can lead to premature death if not corrected or treated on time. That is why the Spanish Association of Self-care (ANEFP) promotes self-care as the key for the prevention of serious diseases [2], but also in the recovery from a mild and transitory illness [40].

In order to achieve these purposes, a series of technology strategies involving CAs have been created by researchers and developers to educate and counsel on the importance of good habits such as self-management of chronic disease [9, 13, 29, 50], health behavior change [8, 19, 34, 55] and education in specific issues [11, 16, 24, 66]. As shown in Table 7.2, the existing literature on these topics is abundant due to the urgent need to raise awareness the role of education for the well-being of the population.

With respect to the self-management of chronic disease, there are some technology strategies that have been developed to allow patients to better manage their health on a daily basis. For example, in 2005, Lesley-Ann Black et al. [13] proposed a remote monitoring system which involves patients with diabetes and co-existing hypertension to participate proactively in the care of their condition. Subsequently, in 2014, Hyekyun Rhee et al. [50] proposed a natural dialogue system to promote asthma self-management, being an aid for adolescents with this condition and their parents. In 2018, Klaassen et al. [29] proposed a platform that integrates a virtual coach to support young patients in diabetes self-management through an educational game. In the same year, Bickmore et al. [9] proposed a virtual agent to advise patients with a chronic heart condition about self-managment of their disease.

TABLE 7.2
Published Studies Related to Conversational Agents for Education and Counseling

Health Domain	First Author, Year	Target Population
Self-management of chronic disease	Timothy W. Bickmore et al., 2018 [9]	People with the chronic heart condition
	Randy Klaassen et al., 2018 [29]	Patients with diabetes
	Hyekyun Rhee et al., 2014 [50]	People with asthma
	Lesley-Ann Black et al., 2005 [13]	Patients with diabetes
Education and counseling about specific issue	Shuo Zhou et al., 2018 [66]	Adolescents
	Paula Gardiner et al., 2013 [24]	Women and mothers
	Roger A. Edwards et al., 2013 [19]	Women and mothers
	Rik Crutzen et al., 2011 [16]	Adolescents
Health behavior change	Timothy W. Bickmore et al., 2013 [11]	All stakeholders
	Christine Lisseti et al., 2013 [34]	All stakeholders
	Daniel Schulman et al., 2011 [55]	All stakeholders
	Timothy W. Bickmore et al., 2005 [8]	Older adults

In all of the above studies, different types of CAs are used to facilitate symptom monitoring, treatment adherence, question-solving and the promotion of healthy habits. These strategies were designed to provide better and increased care to those who need it, due to the increasing number of patients with chronic diseases. In terms of qualitative results, through an interview, all the studies evaluated how participants felt after their experience with the respective CA. The participants appreciated the level of personalisation [13], considering it was an attractive and convenient option to facilitate self-management [50]. In the same way, in some cases, during the study participants demonstrated improvements in their conditions by decreasing the frequency with which symptoms occurred [9, 50].

Subsequently, with regard to education and counseling about a specific issue, the existing literature is recent because this area emerged a short while ago to complement the efforts of health professionals to educate and support on certain issues. As is the case of Crutzen et al. [16], who in 2011 proposed a chatbot that answered questions about sex, drugs, and alcohol. In 2013, Edwards et al. [19] presented an interactive agent that provided breastfeeding information and support to mothers interested in breastfeeding. In the same year, Gardiner et al. [24] developed an animated character to promote the concept of preconception care, improving the health of women and mitigating risk factors prior to pregnancy. Lastly, in 2018, Zhou et al. [66] proposed a virtual agent to advise people with alcohol problems about their situation.

Although the above-mentioned studies vary in their target population, the aim for which they were designed is the same. The purpose is to help patients resolve their questions by allowing them to develop their own understanding of the problem and what can be done about it. As to the qualitative results of these four studies, just three of them measure the level of satisfaction with the CA. Two of these use a 7-point satisfaction survey [19, 24] and one uses 5-point Likert Scale [16]. Despite this difference in evaluation, mean overall satisfaction with the CA was high. The patients were very satisfied and, additionally, the CAs were perceived as a faster and anonymous tool to seek reliable information [16].

Last but not least, there were four documents found in the literature related to health behavior change. All of these are aimed at encouraging patients to change their health behavior due to bad habits that can diminish the quality and duration of patients' lives. For these reasons, researchers have developed some technology strategies based on evidence, which are described below. In 2005, Bickmore et al. [8] proposed a relational agent for older adults who would play the role of physical activity advisor. Later, in 2011, Schulman et al. [55] presented a virtual agent to promote physical exercise, improving people's motivation and confidence through dialogue. In 2013, Lisseti et al. [34] proposed a customized virtual agent to encourage the reduction of alcohol consumption in problem drinkers through brief motivational interventions. And finally, in the same year, Bickmore et al. [11] proposed an automated agent to promote both physical activity and fruit and vegetable consumption through a series of conversations.

By conducting a 7-point satisfaction survey [55] and a Godspeed questionnaire [6, 34], it could be concluded that the CAs were accepted and liked. These results are very promising, especially since in some cases, the intervention of the CAs was effective in achieving an increase in physical activity and in the consumption of fruit and vegetables [11].

In general, the results of these studies suggest that the use of CAs in education and counseling has a positive impact on the population, as it provides users with appropriate feedback or advice for health promotion, disease prevention and care during illness.

7.3.2 Rehabilitation

According to the WHO, rehabilitation is a set of interventions needed when a person is experiencing limitations in everyday functioning due to ageing or a health condition, including chronic diseases or disorders, injuries or traumas [45]. Examples of limitations in functioning include difficulties in having relationships, communicating, and moving around, among others [5]. Based on the foregoing, the area of rehabilitation is a very broad domain that includes several specialties, among which are (i) communication skills rehabilitation, (ii) speech and language therapy, (iii) physical rehabilitation and (iv) psychological rehabilitation.

At present, the need of rehabilitation is largely unmet due to, in many low- and middle-income countries, a lack of trained professionals to provide rehabilitation services, with less than 10 skilled practitioners per 1 million population [45]. That is why researchers and developers support the idea of using CAs to supplement the shortage of staff in healthcare centers. As shown in Table 7.3, CAs have been used to support the rehabilitation processes of people with Austim Spectrum Disorder (ASD) [59, 64, 65], neurological conditions [27, 52, 62], mobility-impairment [17, 57] and psychological trauma [53], which represent a large percentage of the total number of people with disabilities.

In relation to the area of communication skills rehabilitation, the literature found has as its target population children with ASD. ASD is a developmental disorder that affects communication and social interaction. In addition, the number of children diagnosed with ASD has been rising dramatically in recent years [64]. Therefore, there are many treatments that can help children acquire new skills and overcome

TABLE 7.3
Published Studies Related to Conversational Agents for Rehabilitation

Health Domain	First Author, Year	Target Population
Communication skills rehab	Hiroki Tanaka et al., 2017 [59]	Children with autism
	Loo Weilun et al., 2011 [64]	Children with autism
Speech and language therapy	David Ireland et al., 2016 [27]	People with neurological conditions
	Sarel vanBuuren et al., 2014 [62]	People with aphasia
	Preben Wik et al., 2009 [65]	Children with autism
Physical rehab	Judith Deutsch et al., 2012 [17]	Individuals post-stroke
Psychological rehab	Albert Rizzo et al., 2011 [53]	Military members

a wide variety of developmental challenges [38]. For example, in 2011, Weilun et al. [64] proposed a virtual agent as an augmentative aid to engage students with ASD in rehabilitative and academic training through virtual games. In the same way, in 2017, Tanaka et al. [59] presented a dialogue system that teaches and trains communication skills in children with autism through interaction with an avatar.

Both studies evaluated the effect of the agent intervention using different strategies. In the first study [64], the impact was evaluated through feedback given by students. Each student interacted with the games for 10 to 15 minutes, and at the end of the interaction, the students were requested to fill up a feeback form (unspecified). All of them expressed acceptance and appreciation for the games and the virtual agent. On the other hand, in the second study [59], the system's effectiveness was evaluated by comparing pre- and post-training scores predicted by the system. The result of this study showed significant improvement in social skills between pre- and post-training, as well as the relationships between the overall social skills and other non-verbal behaviors.

Subsequently, with regard to speech and language therapy, there are several populations of interest, due to there being many reasons why speech can be affected. For example, as a result of suffering from neurological diseases [27], aphasia [62] and ASD [65], children and adults may experience speaking and communication problems. That is why researchers have developed rehabilitation strategies to improve the quality of life of people suffering from these limitations. As is the case of Wik et al. [65], who in 2009 described an embodied conversational agent for language learning in children and younger. The agent takes the role of a teacher who guides, encourages and gives feedback. In 2014 vanBuuren et al. [62] proposed a virtual therapist for delivering speech and language therapy to people with aphasia by visibly exemplifying speech. And finally, in 2016, Ireland et al. [27] tested an artificial agent to converse with the user, and in turn measure voice and communication outcomes during the daily life of the user. This last development was aimed at people with Parkinson's disease and dementia, who have difficulties in language and communication.

Three different strategies are used by each of the studies to measure their effect. For example, in the first study [65], a request was sent to all the people who had used the agent to fill out a questionnaire in order to get some qualitative feedback. All questions were multiple choice with the range from 1 (I do not agree at all) to 5 (I totally agree). On average, the scores were over 3.29, which led to the conclusion that the agent has been well received by the people. In the second study [62], no assessment was made regarding perception or acceptability. But as a conclusion, the study indicated that for persons with aphasia, receiving treatment supported by a virtual therapist can lead to faster learning. Finally, related to the third study [27], participants were given time to speak with an agent and then subsequently asked to share their experiences. The overall impression of use of the agent was positive, and participants also identified technical problems such as processing speed.

On the other hand, concerning the physical rehabilitation, there are some examples that take advantage of the non-human characteristics of CAs to repeatedly exemplify exercises without getting tired. Given the above, CAs are being used as a potential tool to support health professionals during physical rehabilitation sessions. As is the case of Deutsch et al. [17] who in 2012 proposed a system to address motor control and fitness deficits in people who have had a stroke. In this study, an avatar was used to exemplify the movement and speed the user had to follow to stay within a safe training range. As a result, all participants attended all scheduled sessions, representing 100% adherence to rehabilitation. In the same way, all participants increased their aerobic capacity as measured by their oxygen consumption.

Finally, in the area of psychological rehabilitation, few studies use CAs possibly due to the complexity of the issues involved in this area. As is the case with Rizzo et al. [53] who in 2011 developed a series of virtual agents to serve as online guides. This project is aimed to motivate users to take the first step and seek information and advice with regard to their health through dialogue. Actually, this project is currently available online [22] so that anyone interested can dialogue with the virtual agents. In fact, the designed CAs can effectively discuss personal self-care concerns by both answering questions and providing guidance.

Overall, the results of these studies suggest that the use of CAs in the rehabilitation area has great potential in motivating and exciting the patients in their recovery process [59]; also the patients prove to be highly receptive of the CA [57]. In conclusion, the use of CAs in rehabilitation could provide new opportunities in order to compensate for the lack of skilled practitioners in some places. Or given the current situation, promote telerehabilitation programs that allow people to continue their rehabilitation processes at home and at a low cost.

7.3.3 Mental Health

According to the WHO, around 450 million people currently suffer from mental disorders, placing these conditions among the leading causes of ill-health and disability worldwide [23]; which is a worrying figure that increases every year, aggravating the situation. That is why mental health has become a major field of action of CAs due to mental illnesses affecting a person's thinking, feeling, behavior or mood, and having a profound impact on day-to-day living and, some cases, mental illness can lead to suicide [4]. For these reasons, most studies in this area are oriented to support the early diagnosis [49] and treatment of mental illnesses [21, 35, 51, 60] as shown in Table 7.4.

TABLE 7.4
Published Studies Related to Conversational Agents for Mental Health

Health Domain	First Author, Year	Target Population
Treating mood disorders	Ameneh Shamekhi et al., 2018 [56]	People with anxiety and depression
	Kathleen Fitzpatrick et al.,2017 [21]	People with anxiety and depression
	Myrthe L. Tielman et al., 2017 [60]	People with post-traumatic stress disorder
Support to diagnostic of mental disorders	Pierre Philip et al., 2017 [49]	People with major depressive disorders

Most mental disorders such as schizophrenia, depression, anxiety, Post-Traumatic Stress Disorder (PTSD), intellectual disabilities and disorders due to drug abuse can be successfully treated; however, more than half of those affected worldwide do not receive treatment. In some cases, stigma, discrimination and neglect prevent care and treatment from reaching people with mental disorders, according to the WHO [41]. For these cases, CAs could be the ideal tool for the support in the diagnosis or treatment of these conditions, becoming the best alternative to address this problem because they can be applied all over the world at a very low cost.

Based on the current evidence, the CAs could be used for the diagnosis of mental disorders and the treatment of these conditions. For the first application mentioned above, CAs act as a support to the health professional through the identification of specific symptoms. As is the case of Philip et al. [49], who in 2017 presented an Embodied Conversational Agent (ECA) to identify specific symptoms related to depression in outpatients. According to experts, a face-to-face clinical interview is the gold standard to diagnose mental disorders. That is why, the researchers developed an agent able to conduct a face-to-face interview, identify specific symptoms and diagnose depression. As a result, patients found the face-to-face interview with the agent very acceptable according to the AES scale. The good level of acceptability suggests that the agent can communicate empathy, elicit patient trust and reduce the feeling of being judged by a human [49]. On the other hand, the validity of the depression diagnosis performed by the agent in comparison with the diagnosis of the psychiatrist was satisfactory. Its specificity was also good irrespective of the severity of the depressive symptoms, so the agent efficiently identified patients with and without depression.

For the treatment of these disorders, the CAs act as an indispensable friend by providing a self-help program until the symptoms improve. Currently, three documents have been found that expose the use of CAs for treating mood disorders, especially for anxiety, depression and PTSD. The first study was proposed in 2017 by Tielman et al. [60] who designed a virtual agent to inform and guide patients with PTSD to recall their memories in a digital diary regaining a sense of control over own life. In that same year, Fitzpatrick et al. [21] proposed a conversational agent to deliver a self-help program for college students who self-identified as having symptoms of anxiety and depression. And later, in 2018, Shamekhi et al. [56] designed a virtual coach to alleviate symptoms related to pain, anxiety, and depression through meditation. Overall, the results of these studies suggest that the use of CAs in this domain breaks down barriers to care such as stigma, prejudice, grief, and fear, among others. Additionally, preliminary evidence speaks favorably of the acceptance of CAs by patients due to their omnipresence and their ability to serve without judgment, unlike humans.

Finally, WHO emphasized that the burden of depression and other mental health conditions is on the rise globally [47] and it is important to continue to create alternatives for a comprehensive and coordinated response to mental disorders [4].

7.3.4 Physical Training

According to the WHO, lack of physical activity has been identified as the fourth largest risk factor for global mortality, accounting for about 6% of deaths worldwide [44].

TABLE 7.5
Published Studies Related to Conversational Agents for Physical Training

Health Domain	First Author, Year	Target Population
Weight management	Cynthia LeRouge et al., 2016 [33]	Adolescents with overweight problem
	Alice Watson et al., 2012 [63]	Adults with overweight problem
Physical activity	Timothy W. Bickmore et al., 2013 [12]	Sedentary older adults
	Terry Ellis et al., 2013 [20]	Persons with Parkinson's disease

In this sense, physical activity is a key factor in prevention of chronic diseases like overweight [44] and, in some cases, in care during degenerative illness such as Parkinson's disease [20].

Performing physical activity has significant health benefits, consequently the development of technological alternatives that promote regular, planned and structured physical exercise could improve the quality of life of the global population. To this end, CAs are a good way to promote physical activity through a series of simulated conversations with users, exemplification of the movements and accompaniment during training sessions.

Based on the existing literature, the main purpose of CAs in this field is to motivate and support users to perfom regular physical exercise, especially in a population that is overweight and has a sedentary lifestyle and motor limitations as shown in Table 7.5. Actually, there are two domains where the intervention of CAs can increase adherence to physical exercise; as a consequence, people can lose weight [33, 63] and manage their physical and physiological conditions [12, 20].

Firstly, in relation to weight loss, the fight against obesity and excessive weight in adolescents and adults requires the development of effective interventions. For example, most treatment guidelines recommend that people who are overweight or obese aim to lose 5 to 10% of their weight to achieve improvements in health [39]. For these reasons, researchers have proposed some strategies to lose weight by increasing physical activity levels. As is the case for Watson et al. [63] who in 2012 proposed a virtual coach that promotes the performance of physical exercise on a regular basis. In the same way, in 2016, LeRouge et al. [33] presented a study to address how avatars can help obese adolescents commit to weight loss.

In the first study [63], the participants reported beneficial changes in their lifestyle, such as exercising more frequently and improving diet and eating habits. In the same way, they were asked specific questions regarding their interactions with the virtual coach: 58% (of total participants) agreed that the coach motivated them to become more active, and 87% reported feeling guilty if they skipped an appointment with the coach. In the second study [33], the adolescents felt great interest in including avatars in their overweight management programs to make it more fun and entertaining. Also, they felt the avatars could reinforce the guidance and support provided by lifestyle modification programs. As a conclusion of both studies, the use of CAs may be a means to increase the engagement of obese adolescents participating in a weight management program.

On the other hand, concerning the management of physical and physiological conditions, the strategies that currently exist are aimed at taking advantage of the potential role of exercise in reducing disabilies in person with Parkinson's disease [20] and creating adherence to exercise in sedentary older adults [12]. Based on the above, it was Ellis et al. who in 2013 proposed a virtual exercise coach to promote daily walking in persons with Parkinson's disease in order to reduce the physical limitations that they present due to their condition. In that same year, Bickmore et al. [12] presented an ECA designed specifically for older adults who are in need of greater mobility, to promote and improve physical activity.

As a result of the first study [20], the level of satisfaction and adherence to the program was assessed. On average, the participants had a mean satisfaction score of 5.6 over 7 (with 7 indicating maximal satisfaction). Besides, they successfully used the virtual coach at home to adhere to a walking program for 1 month, demonstrating the initial feasibility of this approach. In the second study [12], the level of satisfaction was assessed through interviews, where participants expressed a high level of satisfaction and acceptability towards the agent. In relation to quantitative results, the number of steps was measured throughout the study, showing significant increases in walking from the first intervention.

All these findings suggest that the use of CAs in physical training may be a useful adjunct to existing automated applications designed to promote physical activity. Furthermore, given the current situation with a global pandemic, the promotion of programs that allow people to exercise at home will make it possible to combat the mental and physical consequences of the COVID-19 quarantine [28].

7.3.5 Palliative Care

The WHO estimates that more than 20 million patients need palliative care each year; about one third of them have cancer, and the rest suffer from degenerative diseases or life-threatening chronic illnesses [40]. That is why, the purpose of palliative care is not only to relieve pain, but also to alleviate the physical, psychosocial and emotional suffering of patients with serious illnesses in their advanced stages and to help the families of these people care for their loved ones [42].

In view of the above, palliative care also is an emerging field in which CAs could intervene to relieve the suffering and worries of those with terminal diseases who do not respond to curative treatments. The current evidence is supported by two studies, which are shown in Table 7.6.

TABLE 7.6
Published Studies Related to Conversational Agents for Palliative Care

Health Domain	First Author, Year	Target Population
Crisis support	Katherine Easton et al., 2019 [18]	People with chronic obstructive pulmonary disease
End-of-life planning	Dina Utami et al., 2017 [61]	Older adults

Based on the literature, there are two domains in the area of palliative care, where CAs can intervene: crisis support and end-of-life planning. Concerning the last one, in 2017, Utami et al. [61] presented a virtual agent that helps people manage symptoms and reduce stress during their last year of life. The study was conducted in a single session, and in order to determine the attitude of participants towards agents, a 12-question questionnaire was conducted on a scale of 1 (very unsatisfied) to 7 (very satisfied). In general, this study demonstrates that older adults react positively to the agent. Similarly, older adults are comfortable discussing these topics with the agent, as they showed a significant reduction in their anxiety state.

On the other hand, in 2018, Easton et al. [18] presented a virtual agent for supporting people with Chronic Obstructive Pulmonary Disease (COPD) by creating a therapeutic relationship between the agent and the user, in particular for crisis support. As a result, this study indicated that the benefits of this low-cost system include increased self-confidence, less social isolation, and better patient awareness of the disease. Clinical gains include fewer acute exacerbations and a decrease in utilization of the conventional healthcare service.

As shown above, the intervention of CAs in this field may involve innumerable benefits and gains, always aimed at improving the quality of life of patients and their families facing life-threatening diseases.

7.4 FUTURE WORKS

As highlighted in the previous section, due to a growing research interest in creating CAs that can attend to people, it is important that researchers and developers of CAs for healthcare delivery understand their limitations in order to improve and explore new features. In the same way, taking into account the studies analyzed and their results, a number of recommendations for future designs and work are presented below.

7.4.1 Limitations

In Section 7.3 it was proved that CAs are being tested and used to provide and collect information related to people's health and, in some cases, provide treatment and counseling services. They are becoming more popular and sophisticated than ever, but their abilities, at least for now, do have significant limitations.

In the majority of cases, CAs are based on speech and may have limited conversations [25], some of the others tend to work in the background providing information when and where needed [51]. Nevertheless, the scope and adaptability of these strategies is limited by the variability of the user preferences, context and noise in the user input. Additionally, most CA applications do not integrate wearable devices being a great limitation because the feedback, advice or assistance provided by the agent is not based on the state of the organism. And as a consequence, the reliability and security of the agent's intervention are affected.

The limitations mentioned above become challenges for CAs for medical applications directly impacting the quality of life and health of people by affecting the way healthcare services are provided. To this end, it would be ideal that CAs have the following characteristics [51]: (i) having spoken, multimodal and multisensorial understanding, (ii) understanding covert signals, (iii) being able to handle basic and complex emotions such as empathy, (iv) being aware of the user's current status, and finally (v) having the ability to carry out a dialogue with a human.

On the other hand, as the intervention of CAs implies direct interaction with human beings, it is important to consider that there are ethical limitations for their widespread use; for example, the appearance and behavior of designed CAs are susceptible to design biases, such as preference for a particular racial or ethnic background. Consequently, their developers must consider data from target population and diverse communities within a population who could be affected by disparities in testing and implementation of these technologies.

7.4.2 Recommendations

Considering the limitations mentioned above, there were a number of recommendations and critical points for future designs and research, as shown below:

> During the design phase, the 24×7 availability of the CA must be taken into account and its potential to provide assistance at exactly the right moment (e.g., just before or after a specific behavior) making it a potentially valuable tool.
>
> Furthermore, during the data analysis phase of an evaluation, the outcomes should be linked to measures of effectiveness, usage, and user experience, to understand if the CA works and why. This is the only way a single evaluation can be valuable.
>
> Whenever possible, the use of wearable devices should be increased such as sensors that measure vitals without the patient being restricted to a bed, in order to provide better healthcare services and greater certainty about the feedback that is being made.
>
> Lastly, to fully understand the effect that the intervention of CAs may generate over time, longitudinal studies need to be performed. Most of the documents studied present results and conclusions from pilot studies or cross-sectional studies, leaving poor evidence of the benefits of long-term intervention of CAs.

7.5 CONCLUSIONS

As an initial observation, one of the advantages of CAs is that they can be replicated easily and affordably to meet demand and, unlike humans, users can access them via Internet at any time and almost anywhere. Additionally, they could potentially be more reliable than humans because they are unaffected by fatigue, exhaustion and cognitive errors. However, despite the potential qualities mentioned above, these technologies have been and are being developed to support health professionals in some specific process rather than replacing them. Therefore, it is essential that the developers of these technologies provide users with sufficient information on the scope, risks, limits and expectations in relation to the use of CAs.

Also, CA developers can design them to have modifiable physical appearance, language and dialect, and other characteristics that match them to a user's cultural background, including race and ethnicity or socioeconomic status. This can help build a relationship with users, contributing positively to adherence to treatments and better health outcomes.

Currently, there are very few studies in the literature that refer to the quantitative results of the intervention of CAs. However, the qualitative results suggest a good user perception that is reflected in increased motivation, willingness and adherence to the process. Although the results presented in this chapter are promising, this research is still at an early stage. Thus, the findings of this work will serve as the basis to promote long-term studies and the integration of wearable devices. It would be valuable to validate these studies in a higher number of participants providing meaningful information, by conducting an appropriate statistical analysis of effectiveness.

Aditionally, it is necessary to highlight the systems that integrate wearable devices with CAs because it allows to enhance application, an option that is widely available and is often inexpensive. This becomes a promising approach to the development of improved health services through the integration of CAs with wearable devices to build systems that are able to deliver medical services with a certain degree of autonomy. As is the case in this chapter, showing evidence of appropriate use and benefits generated by a CA helps address concerns about technology and potentially accelerates its adoption.

REFERENCES

[1] Critical appraisal skills programme. CASP checklist: 11 questions to help you make sense of a case control study. https://casp-uk.net/wp-content/uploads/2018/01/CASP-Case-Control-Study-Checklist-2018.pdf, 2018.

[2] Araceli Aguilar, Julio Cansino, Noemi Giné, M. Dolores Matas, Marta Miras, and Luís Valdayo. Información sobre la seguridad en asma, diabetes e hipertensión de las especialidades farmacéuticas sin receta, según distintas fuentes terciarias. *Seguim farmacoter*, 1(3): 115–119, 2003.

[3] AliveCor. Kardia mobile de AliveCor. https://www.alivecor.com/ifus/kardiamobile/02LB53.1-es.pdf, 2017.

[4] American Psychiatric Association. What is depression? https://www.psychiatry.org/patients-families/depression/what-is-depression, 2017.

[5] Skye Barbic, Susan Bartlett, and Nancy Mayo. Emotional vitality: Concept of importance for rehabilitation. *Archives of physical medicine and rehabilitation*, 94(8):1547–1554, 2013.

[6] Christoph Bartneck, Elizabeth Croft, and Dana Kulic. Measurement instruments for the anthropomorphism, animacy, likeability, perceived intelligence, and perceived safety of robots. *International journal of social robotics*, 1(1):71–81, 2009.

[7] Martin Beveridge and John Fox. Automatic generation of spoken dialogue from medical plans and ontologies. *Journal of biomedical informatics*, 39(5):482–99, 2006.

[8] Timothy W. Bickmore, Lisa Caruso, Kerri Clough-Gorr, and Tim Heeren. "It's just like you talk to a friend". Relational agents for older adults. *Interacting with computers*, 17:711–735, 2005.

[9] Timothy W. Bickmore, Everlyne Kimani, Ha Trinh, Alexandra Pusateri, Michael K. Paasche-Orlow, and Jared W. Magnani. Managing chronic conditions with a smartphone-based conversational virtual agent. *Proceedings of the 18th International Conference on Intelligent Virtual Agents*, pages 119–124, November 2018.

[10] Timothy W. Bickmore, Dan Mauer, and Thomas Brown. Context awareness in a handheld exercise agent. *Pervasive and mobile computing*, 5(3):226–235, 2009.

[11] Timothy W. Bickmore, Daniel Schulman, and Candace Sidner. Automated interventions for multiple health behaviors using conversational agents. *Patient education and counseling*, 92(2), 142–148, 2013.

[12] Timothy W. Bickmore, Rebecca A. Silliman, Kerrie Nelson, Debbie M. Cheng, Michael Winter, Lori Henault, and Michael K. Paasche-Orlow. A randomized controlled trial of an automated exercise coach for older adults. *Journal of the American Geriatrics Society*, 61(10), 1676–1683, 2013.
[13] L.A. Black, Michael Mctear, Norman Black, Roy Harper, and M. Lemon. Appraisal of a conversational artefact and its utility in remote patient monitoring. *18th IEEE Symposium on Computer-Based Medical Systems, pages* 506–508, Dublin, Ireland, June 23–24, 2005.
[14] Justine Cassell, Joseph Sullivan, Scott Prevost, and Elizabeth Churchill. Embodied Conversational Agents. The MIT Press, Cambridge, MA, https://mitpress.mit.edu/books/embodied-conversational-agents, 2000.
[15] Indranil Chakraborty and Prasenjit Maity. Covid-19 outbreak: Migration, effects on society, global environment and prevention. *Science of the total environment*, 728:138882, August 1, 2020.
[16] Rik Crutzen, Gjalt-Jorn Peters, Sarah Portugal, Erwin Fisser, and Jacob Jorne. An artificially intelligent chat agent that answers adolescents' questions related to sex, drugs, and alcohol: An exploratory study. *Journal of adolescent health: official publication of the society for adolescent medicine*, 48(5):514–519, 2011.
[17] Judith Deutsch, Mary Myslinski, R. Ranky, Mark Sivak, Constantinos Mavroidis, and Jeffrey Lewis. Fitness improved for individuals post-stroke after virtual reality augmented cycling training. *ICDVRAT Conference*, September 1, 2012.
[18] Katherine Easton, Stephen Potter, Remi Bec, Matthew Bennion, Heidi Christensen, Cheryl Grindell, Bahman Mirheidari, Scott Weich, Luc Witte, Daniel Wolstenholme, and Mark Hawley. A virtual agent to support individuals living with physical and mental comorbidities: Co-design and acceptability testing. *Journal of medical internet research*, 21(5): 2019.
[19] Roger Edwards, Timothy Bickmore, Lucia Jenkins, Mary Foley, and Justin Manjourides. Use of an interactive computer agent to support breastfeeding. *Maternal and child health journal*, 17(10): 1961–1968, 2013.
[20] Terry Ellis, Nancy Latham, Tamara Deangelis, Cathi Thomas, Marie Saint-Hilaire, and Timothy Bickmore. Feasibility of a virtual exercise coach to promote walking in community-dwelling persons with Parkinson disease. *American journal of physical medicine & rehabilitation/Association of Academic Physiatrists*, 92(6), 2013.
[21] Kathleen Kara Fitzpatrick, Alison Darcy, and Molly Vierhile. Delivering cognitive behavior therapy to young adults with symptoms of depression and anxiety using a fully automated conversational agent (woebot): A randomized controlled trial. *JMIR mental health*, 4(2): e19, 2017.
[22] Institute for Creative Technologies-University of Southern California. Prototype of simcoach beta. https://www.simcoach.org/, 2013.
[23] Silvana Galderisi, Andreas Heinz, Marianne Kastrup, Julian Beezhold, and Norman Sartorius. Toward a new definition of mental health. *World psychiatry*, 14(2):231–233, 2015.
[24] Paula Gardiner, Megan Hempstead, Lazlo Ring, Timothy Bickmore, Leanne Yinusa-Nyahkoon, Huong Trần, Paashe-Orlow M., Karla Damus, and Brian Jack. Reaching women through health information technology: The Gabby preconception care system. *American journal of health promotion*, 27(3 suppl):eS11–eS20, 2013.
[25] Marti A. Hearst. "Natural" search user interfaces. *Communications of the ACM*, 54(11):60–67, 2011.
[26] Eva Hudlicka. Virtual affective agents and therapeutic games, In *Artificial Intelligence in Behavioral and Mental Health Care*, Edited by David Luxton, pages 81–115, Elsevier, 2016.

[27] David Ireland, Christina Atay (née Knuepffer), Jacki Liddle, Dana Bradford, Helen Lee, Olivia Rushin, Thomas Mullins, Daniel Angus, Janet Wiles, Simon McBride, and Adam Vogel. Hello Harlie: Enabling speech monitoring through chat-bot conversations. *Studies in health technology and informatics*, 227:55–60, 2016.

[28] David Jiménez-Pavón, Ana Carbonell-Baeza, and Carl Lavie. Physical exercise as therapy to fight against the mental and physical consequences of COVID-19 quarantine: Special focus in older people. *Progress in cardiovascular diseases*, 63(3): 386–388, 2020.

[29] Randy Klaassen, Kim C.M. Bul, Rieks Op den Akker, Gert Jan van der Burg, Pamela M., and Pierpaolo Di Bitonto. Design and evaluation of a pervasive coaching and gamification platform for young diabetes patients. *Sensors*, 18(2):402, 2018.

[30] Lean Kramer, Silke ter Stal, Bob Mulder, Emely Vet, and Lex van Velsen. Developing embodied conversational agents for coaching people in a healthy lifestyle: Scoping review. *Journal of medical internet research*, 22(2): 2020.

[31] Liliana Laranjo, Adam Dunn, Huong Ly Tong, A. Baki Kocaballi, Jessica Chen, Rabia Bashir, Didi Surian, Blanca Gallego, Farah Magrabi, Annie Lau, and Enrico Coiera. Conversational agents in healthcare: A systematic review. *Journal of the American Medical Informatics Association,*25(9): 1248-1258, 2018.

[32] Sven Laumer, Christian Maier, and Fabian Tobias Gubler. Chatbot acceptance in healthcare: Explaining user adoption of conversational agents for disease diagnosis. In *Proceedings of the 27th European Conference on Information Systems (ECIS)*, Stockholm & Uppsala, Sweden, June 8–14, 2019.

[33] Cynthia Lerouge, Kathryn Dickhut, Christine Lisetti, Savitha Sangameswaran, and Toree Malasanos. Engaging adolescents in a computer-based weight management program: Avatars and virtual coaches could help. *Journal of the American Medical Informatics Association*, 23(1):19–28, 2016.

[34] Christine Lisetti, Reza Amini, Ugan Yasavur, and N. Rishe. I can help you change! An empathic virtual agent delivers behavior change health interventions. *ACM Transactions on Management Information Systems*, 19, December 2013.

[35] Gale Lucas, Albert Rizzo, Jonathan Gratch, Stefan Scherer, Giota Stratou, Jill Boberg, and Louis-Philippe Morency. Reporting mental health symptoms: Breaking down barriers to care with virtual human interviewers. *Frontiers in robotics and AI*, 4:51, October 2017.

[36] Martin Luerssen and Tim Hawke. Virtual agents as a service: Applications in healthcare in*Proceedings of the 18th International Conference on Intelligent Virtual Agents*, pages 107–112, November 2018.

[37] Michael McTear, Zoraida Callejas, and David Griol. *The Conversational Interface: Talking to Smart Devices*. Springer Publishing Company, Inc., 1st edition, 2016.

[38] Scott M. Myers and Chris Plauché Johnson. Management of children with autism spectrum disorders. *Pediatrics*, 120(5):1162–1182, 2007.

[39] National Institutes of Health. Benefits of moderate weight loss in people with obesity. https://www.nih.gov/news-events/nih-research-matters/benefits-moderate-weight-loss-people-obesit,2016.

[40] World Health Organization. Who definition of palliative care. https://www.who.int/cancer/palliative/definition/en/, n.d.

[41] World Health Organization. Mental disorders affect one in four people. https://www.who.int/whr/2001/media_centre/press_release/en/, 2001.

[42] World Health Organization. Primer Atlas Mundial de las necesidades de cuidados paliativos no atendidas. https://www.who.int/mediacentre/news/releases/2014/palliative-care-20140128/es/, 2014.

[43] World Health Organization. Noncommunicable diseases. https://www.who.int/news-room/fact-sheets/detail/noncommunicable-diseases, 2018.

[44] World Health Organization. Physical activity. https://www.who.int/news-room/fact-sheets/detail/physical-activity, 2018.
[45] World Health Organization. Rehabilitation. https://www.who.int/news-room/fact-sheets/detail/rehabilitation, 2019.
[46] World Health Organization. Coronavirus disease (COVID-19) pandemic. https://www.who.int/emergencies/diseases/novel-coronavirus-2019, 2020.
[47] World Health Organization. Depression. https://www.who.int/news-room/fact-sheets/detail/depression, 2020.
[48] Shyamal Patel, Hyung-Soon Park, Paolo Bonato, Leighton Chan, and Mary Rodgers. A review of wearable sensors and systems with application in rehabilitation. *Journal of neuroengineering and rehabilitation*, 9:21, 2012.
[49] Pierre Philip, Jean-Arthur Micoulaud-Franchi, Patricia Sagaspe, et al. Virtual human as a new diagnostic tool, a proof of concept study in the field of major depressive disorders. *Scientific reports*, 7, 42656, 2017.
[50] Hyekyun Rhee, James Allen, Jennifer Mammen, and Mary Swift. Mobile phone-based asthma self-management aid for adolescents (mASMAA): A feasibility study. *Patient preference and adherence*, 8:63–72, January 2014.
[51] Giuseppe Riccardi. Towards healthcare personal agents. In *RFMIR '14: Proceedings of the 2014 Workshop on Roadmapping the Future of Multimodal Interaction Research Including Business Opportunities and Challenges*, page 53–56, New York, NY, USA, 2014.
[52] Laurel Riek and Peter Robinson. Using robots to help people habituate to visible disabilities. In *Proceedings of IEEE International Conference on Rehabilitation Robotics*, 2011:5975453, 2011.
[53] Albert Rizzo, Belinda Lange, J. Buckwalter, Eric Forbell, J. Kim, K. Sagae, J. Williams, Joann Difede, Barbara Rothbaum, Greg Reger, Thomas Parsons, and P. Kenny. An intelligent virtual human system for proving healthcare information and support, *Studies in Health Technology and Informatics*, 163:503–509, 2011.
[54] John Robinson. *Likert Scale*, pages 3620–3621. Springer Netherlands, Dordrecht, 2014.
[55] Daniel Schulman, Timothy Bickmore, and Candace Sidner. An intelligent conversational agent for promoting long-term health behavior change using motivational interviewing. AI and Health Communication, Papers from the 2011 AAAI Spring Symposium, Technical Report SS-11-01, Stanford, CA, USA, March 21–23, 2011.
[56] Ameneh Shamekhi and Timothy Bickmore. Breathe deep: A breath-sensitive interactive meditation coach. *PervasiveHealth '18: Proceedings of the 12th EAI International Conference on Pervasive Computing Technologies for Healthcare*, pages 108–117, May 2018.
[57] Ameneh Shamekhi, Ha Trinh, Timothy Bickmore, Tamara DeAngelis, Theresa Ellis, Bethlyn Houlihan, and Nancy Latham. A virtual self-care coach for individuals with spinal cord injury. *Assets '16: Proceedings of the 18th International ACM SIGACCESS Conference on Computers and Accessibility*, pages 327–328, October 2016.
[58] Valerie Smith, Declan Devane, Cecily Begley, and Mike Clarke. Methodology in conducting a systematic review of systematic review of healthcare interventions. *BMC medical research methodology*, 11:15, 2011.
[59] Hiroki Tanaka, Hideki Negoro, Hidemi Iwasaka, and Satoshi Nakamura. Embodied conversational agents for multimodal automated social skills training in people with autism spectrum disorders. *PLOS ONE*, 12(8):1–15, 2017.
[60] Myrthe Tielman, Mark Neerincx, Rafael Bidarra, Kybartas Ben, and Willem-Paul Brinkman. A therapy system for post-traumatic stress disorder using a virtual agent and virtual storytelling to reconstruct traumatic memories. *Journal of medical systems*, 41, 125, 2017.

[61] Dina Utami, Timothy Bickmore, Asimina Nikolopoulou, and Michael Paasche-Orlow. Talk about death: End of life planning with a virtual agent. In Beskow, J. et al. (eds), *Intelligent Virtual Agents*, pages 441–450, 2017.

[62] Sarel Van Vuuren and Leora R. Cherney. A virtual therapist for speech and language therapy. *Intelligent Virtual Agents*, 8637: 438–448, January 2014.

[63] Alice Watson, Timothy Bickmore, Abby Cange, Ambar Kulshreshtha, and Joseph Kvedar. An internet-based virtual coach to promote physical activity adherence in overweight adults: Randomized controlled trial. *Journal of medical Internet research*, 14:(1), 2012.

[64] L. Weilun, M. R. Elara, and E. M. A. Garcia. Virtual game approach for rehabilitation in autistic children. In *2011 8th International Conference on Information, Communications Signal Processing*, pages 1–6, 2011.

[65] Preben Wik and Anna Hjalmarsson. Embodied conversational agents in computer assisted language learning. *Speech communication*, 51:1024–1037, 2009.

[66] Shuo Zhou, Timothy Bickmore, Amy Rubin, Catherine Yeksigian, Molly Sawdy, and Steven Simon. User gaze behavior while discussing substance use with a virtual agent, in *IVA '18: Proceedings of the 18th International Conference on Intelligent Virtual Agents*, pages 353–354, November 2018.

8 Role of Big Data in e-Healthcare Application for Managing a Large Amount of Data

Meenu Gupta[1]*, Dr. Rachna Jain*[2]*,*
Rachit Singhal[3]*, and Jaspreet Singh*[4]
[1,4]Chandigarh University, Chandigarh, India
[2,3]Bharati Vidyapeeth's College of Engineering, Delhi, India
[1,2,3,4]Department of Computer Science and Engineering

CONTENTS

8.1 Introduction 137
8.1.1 Tabulating Machine 138
8.1.2 Manual Analysis 138
8.1.3 Material Requirement Planning System 138
8.1.4 Pre-Determined Reports 139
8.1.5 Excel Files 139
8.1.6 Databases 139
8.2 Advanced Techniques Used for Managing Large Amounts of Data 140
8.2.1 NoSql 140
8.2.2 Hadoop 143
8.2.3 Spark 145
8.2.4 Pig 148
8.2.5 MapReduce 150
8.2.6 Kafka 154
8.2.7 Hive 159
8.3 Big Data in e-Healthcare 160
8.4 Conclusion 161
References 162

8.1 INTRODUCTION

In the old times, different techniques were used to handle the large amount of data that was being generated. However, these methods were not ideal for the task. These techniques along with their shortcomings and limitations are discussed in this section. There are numerous limitations to Big Data [25]. One research focussed on variety [33] as opposed to velocity and volume. Further, more attention has been given to pre-analysis and post-analysis than analysis itself. Storing such a large amount of data is a key issue as well. In one of the studies, the authors proposed [28] different methods for storing Big Data that is being generated every day from various resources. Starting from hard drives then moving up to optical drives, storage devices are insufficient to hold such a large amount of data. Until now, Cloud services have been used to cope with this situation. Also, there is a trade-off between storage and performance as discussed below:

8.1.1 Tabulating Machine

Dating back to the 1800s, the tabulating machine, built by Herman Hollerith, was one of the first few devices used for summarizing data. The machine was capable of reading data from punched cards and summarizing the data stored on those cards. However, since this machine required data to be punched onto cards, only a limited number of people used the machine. Furthermore, since punched cards are no longer used to store data, these machines are obsolete.

8.1.2 Manual Analysis

Before the advent of Hadoop and R, developers had to manually rummage through the data to find patterns and analyse the data. This process was called Manual Analysis. It was considered one of the most basic methods for analysing data, since it did not require any special software or hardware for data analysis. However, it had various shortcomings:

- Firstly, the developers had to fetch data from different formats. Fetching data can be a very tricky task when the data is stored on different systems having different formats for storing data.
- Secondly, the data could also be inconsistent. It was the task of the developer to go through the data, and find and remove any inconsistencies in the data.
- Thirdly, multiple passes were required to gain full insight into the system which allowed the users to properly analyze data.

8.1.3 Material Requirement Planning System

The Material Requirement Planning (MRP) system performed a specific task and proved to be very complex for a novice user to operate. These systems were designed for three main tasks:

- To ensure proper availability of items.
- To maintain the least number of items in the inventory.
- To plan various activities like manufacturing, delivery and purchasing.

Also, they required structured, accurate data to work on which can be time consuming to generate.

8.1.4 Pre-determined Reports

In the early 1970s, Extract Programs were created to generate reports having a pre-determined template and required information. These programs extracted data from a pre-determined source and created the report using the data as shown in Figure 8.1. These programs could be generated with the click of a button having updated information. But, the template and the source of the information were fixed. Also, these reports could not predict patterns and future values.

8.1.5 Excel Files

Excel provides various features for data analysis like sorting data, data filters, formatting data and many more. In addition to these features, using Excel to represent data graphically is also very simple. All of these features make Excel an ideal choice for data analysis. However, Excel has various shortcomings:

- Excel is unable to handle Big Data of petabyte order.
- Excel does not support unstructured data like media and image files.
- Excel works with past data and is capable of creating graphs using that data. However, it cannot make future predictions.

8.1.6 Databases

A database is used to store data in the form of relational tables. Structured queries can be used to extract data from these databases. Features like Functions and Triggers allow the user to attach special functionality to the queries. Despite having all these advantages, databases are unable to properly process Big Data due to the following:

- Databases allow only structured data to be stored and analysed and cannot be used for unstructured data.
- Databases are Online Transaction Processing (OLTP) tools. Hence, they are designed to store data that is less in volume and is updated regularly. On the other hand, data analysis deals with data which is abundant and is updated sparsely.

Now come modern-day technologies which have proved their existence in every domain providing up to the mark functionalities to users. These technologies are

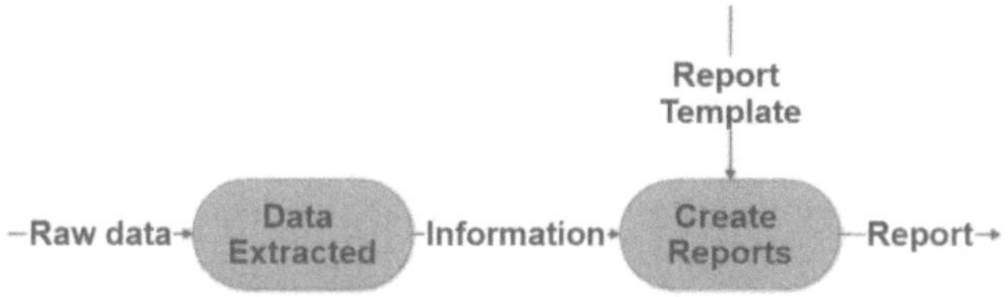

FIGURE 8.1 Pre-determined reports.

not specific to a particular section of society, rather they are targeted by individuals for development and research purposes and also by enterprises around the world to manage their large amount data. These technologies provide full support in analysing these large data sets and gleaning fruitful information from them. Different types of research views related to the area of Big Data and its different applications are discussed in [1] where the authors discussed applications (i.e., CC, IoT, BDA) used as emerging technologies in the field of computation and storage which mainly plays an efficient and effective role in the field of healthcare systems. Further in [2], the authors proposed a new system using Hadoop (i.e., MapReduce, Spark), Cloud infrastructure, monitoring agents to enhance the processing by splitting and processing data streams concurrently. This field is not limited to these technologies. It can be viewed from a data mining perspective as well. Various algorithms are designed to handle data and to generate appropriate results. In [12], the authors proposed a HACE theorem which is used to depict the features of the Big Data Revolution and its processing model in respect to data mining.

8.2 ADVANCED TECHNIQUES USED FOR MANAGING LARGE AMOUNTS OF DATA

From a historical point of view, the amount of data was small and it was easy to manage, as it related to health, environment, or population. But, in the present time due to the increasing number of the population, data increased automatically. To manage huge amounts of data, Cloud computing techniques came into the picture. Due to the pitfalls of cloud computing, industries (or companies) moved to Big Data techniques. In this section, Big Data techniques will be described in detail.

8.2.1 NoSql

Using the orthodox Relational Database Management System (RDBMS) approach is not considered to be beneficial for the rising amount of data which in turn earns the name badge of "Big Data". In relational models, data is organized in a highly well-structured manner, but with the variety in data that is being produced every day, this approach requires some refinement to adjust to variations in the data trends and to provide functionality to users accordingly. NoSql, or Not Only SQL, comes into the picture which can adapt itself to various situations of data, providing extensive scalability and high performance to users. NoSql databases are unstructured in nature thus eradicating the problem of coping with the variations in data trends. It uses the concept of distributed processing where data is stored across multiple nodes or even servers, and results are compiled combining results from all of them.

Using this approach increases the efficiency of computing, reduces time and space complexity, puts less burden on a single system, prevents data loss, etc. Cloud technology is used every day to provide extensive functionality to users and also to cut the hardware costs, maintenance costs, etc. Cloud Computing is a powerful and secure mechanism, but with great functionality comes bigger responsibility. Its presence can be surely felt in every domain these days, and also using Cloud technology in Big Data is not left behind. Most of the Cloud service providers use Big Data with the NoSql approach for maintaining their databases.

In one study, the author described [6] data management research challenges for Big Data and Cloud such as Approximate Results, Data Privacy, Enterprise Data Enrichment with web, Data exploration to enable Deep Analytics, and social media. Organizations across the world strive hard to save big on every transaction they are involved in and to maximize profits. So, does it mean that introduction of this dynamic approach over the past technology will shift the market towards the newly introduced approach? The answer here is simple, in the long term yes, and in the short term not so much. People who have invested a lot of money in building up the infrastructure based upon previous technologies might not have to suffer losses, as these structures are literally the backbone of their organizations, and completely shutting down the whole system to migrate to a new one is not a beneficial option at the present time. One of the critical situations that users face today is which database approach to go with, i.e. SQL or NoSql, so that their needs are completely fulfilled. The SQL approach has surely ruled the past decades providing uniformity and easy functionality, but as the advancements in other domains are happening, Big Data is not left behind in this race. Before NoSql came into the picture, huge record databases needed to be maintained which were difficult to maintain. Inducing business intelligence is another important, as well as necessary, factor for any technology to gain importance. MapReduce is used to implement large amounts of data. A study [9], concluded that in the past four years Google implemented (>10 thousand) MapReduce which is executed on Google clusters to process data (>20 petabytes) per day.

In [31], the authors discussed the use of Big Data and utilization of its methods in the business (i.e., online at the global level) field. With this smart application, people can share their information any time and any place. Revolution came into the industry with the development of Hadoop, and with this revolution older technologies started fading away. The biggest advancement in Hadoop was that it was based on distributed computing. Whole networks were divided into master and slave nodes which enhanced the computing power of a system. Due to similarity in terminology of both Hadoop and NoSql, a buzz was created in the tech industry as both can hand-in-hand provide extensive features with ease. NoSql databases can be of different forms like graph stores, object databases, XML databases, Grid and Cloud, document database, key-value pairs or wide-column stores. These databases do not follow any strict schema design and are therefore suitable for Big Data. One more thing emerges when someone deals with Big Data, i.e., how to scale up the processing to manage the data arriving at faster rates. If someone goes with the relational database concept to manage this much data and that too with many variations, then in some way or another results that will be generated will be either erroneous or incomplete, or any unwanted situation may arise such as system failure, data corruption, etc. NoSql does not follow Atomicity, Consistency, Isolation and Durability (ACID) properties as seen in the case of an SQL approach. When a user submits a query to be operated upon a database, priority is to get the result as soon as possible putting aside the importance of getting the right answer. Therefore, NoSql possesses a weak consistency.

Privacy is also a major factor which decides the performance of any technology. In [22], the authors discussed the need for privacy integration and awareness about security in Big Data platforms. Further, they discussed issues related to the framework which supports privacy integrity access control features in Big Data platforms. There are numerous applications developed using NoSQL approach. The role of Big Data in road transport policies (i.e., Europe) is further discussed [13]. Next, a Cloud computing technique with Big Data was used to analyse the performance of Smart Grids so that customer cost will be reduced in managing data over network [15]. Recommendation and prediction systems are also mostly based on the NoSQL approach. In [17] the authors proposed a personalized contents recommendation service using Big Data which used a small sample so that it accurately predicts the user's preference. It predicts using Big Data with a variety of user information. In another work [18], a model was proposed for analysing and monitoring traffic over the Internet to enhance the quality which is used to promote online investments. Sensor devices are frequently used these days. Data is generated from these devices as well. In [20], the authors summarized the expansion of sensors in Big Data systems (in urban environments), including for assisted living, air pollution monitoring, intelligent transportation, and disaster management systems. With the rapid expansion of fully sequenced and animated plant genomes, plant science has benefitted from next gen sequencing. Authors proposed [26] mechanisms for studying the transcription control of various species using Big Data. Dynamics of life is also studied of various genomes. With a powerful tool (Big Data) in hand, the future can also be predicted. In another application [29], the authors proposed a wind turbine condition monitoring system in which increasing volumes of data are being captured and stored termed as Big Data. The system's capability of capturing huge amounts of data led to the necessity of using enhanced data handling techniques.

It can be clearly observed that for the big techies like Microsoft, IBM, SAP and others, the trend has shifted towards the NoSql approach.

Advantages of NoSql

- Economical
- Big Data applications
- Less support required from database administrator
- Scalable and reliable
- Flexible data models

Disadvantages of NoSql

- Less mature
- Less support
- Analytics and business intelligence issues
- Administration is difficult
- Fewer expert people

This does not mean that using an SQL approach will lead to losses, but the ball is definitely in NoSQL's court, proving its edge over the RDBMS approach.

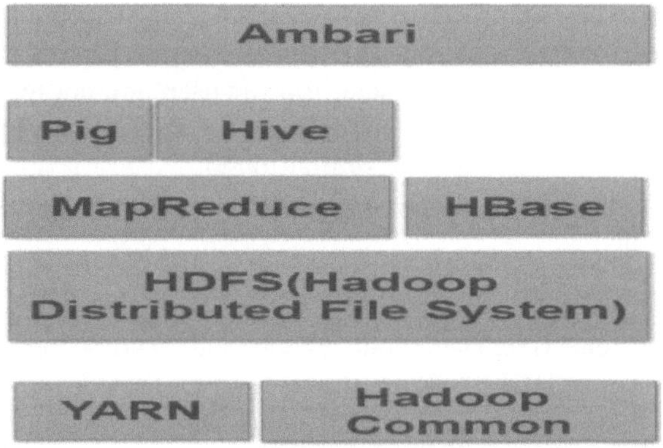

FIGURE 8.2 Hadoop architecture.

8.2.2 Hadoop

Hadoop is a framework written in Java language and is freely available online. It is founded by Doug Cutting and Mike Cafarella, which originated from a paper that was published in October 2003 titled "Google File System". It was named Hadoop by Cutting after his son's toy elephant. Initially, Hadoop contained only MapReduce for data processing. With the development of new modules, Hadoop has become an ecosystem of various data processing technologies like MapReduce, Pig, Hive, etc.

Figure 8.2 shows the architecture of Hadoop which is adequate for storing huge amounts of data in Hadoop Distributed File System (HDFS) and processing using various programming models like MapReduce, Pig, etc. [16].

The Apache Hadoop framework modules are described below:

- **Hadoop Common:** It consists of all Java libraries and other functions required for the basic running of Hadoop and other Hadoop utilities. Hence, it is composed of various Java Archive (JAR) files.
- **YARN** (Yet Another Resource Negotiator): It is a cluster management technology in Hadoop. It has three components namely Resource Manager, Node Manager and Application Manager.
- **HDFS:** It is the main storage in Hadoop. It ensures reliable storage of data by storing a copy of the data on multiple locations.
- **HBase:** It is found at the top of HDFS. It is a column-oriented database which can be used to store and retrieve the data from HDFS. Compared to HDFS, it provides faster lookup and it provides random access to data.
- **MapReduce:** The main functionality of MapReduce is to process data in two ways (i.e., Map and Reduce), and it is developed by Google. Role of Map is to convert the data into intermediate pairs of values or keys, whereas Reduce uses this intermediate data to produce the final result.
- **Pig:** Pig is a tool used to analyse big data sets. Pig contains a programming language called Pig-Latin to access and manipulate data. Furthermore, User Defined Functions (UDFs) in Pig allow users to integrate function written in different languages like Java and Jython.

- **Hive:** In the beginning, Hive was originated by Facebook and later by Apache Software Foundation. The functioning of Hive is similar to Pig, i.e., it is a tool for analysis of data. But the users are not required to learn a completely new language to manipulate the data. Hive uses Hive Query Language (HQL) which is very similar to SQL.
- **Ambari:** It provides a simple and secure platform to manage the entire Hadoop setup.

HDFS plays a very significant role in the successful functionality of Hadoop with three main components (i.e., Data Node, Name Node, and Secondary Name Node). Some of the features of HDFS [43] are the following:

- It uses a master-slave architecture as shown in Figure 8.3, where one system (master node) controls the storage of data on all the other systems (slave nodes).
- It uses low cost commodity hardware to store data.
- It stores data in the form of blocks. The default size of the block is 64 MB or 128 MB. But this can be changed according to the user's preference.
- All the read and write operation on data is done by Data Nodes.
- It has built-in servers of Name Node and Data Nodes that help the user check the status of the cluster.

Hadoop works as a master-slave architecture for storing and accessing data where Name Nodes act as the master and Data Nodes act as the slave. In [19], the authors give a detailed study of Big Data Hadoop and its workings. Further, significance of Hadoop with its classification is also discussed in detail. A multi-node Hadoop Cluster can be set up using the following procedure: Virtual Box could be used to host Ubuntu version 16.04 virtual machines. After installing Hadoop on master and slave nodes, Hadoop services will start with start-all.sh and will be verified with jps commands.

When a query is submitted in Hadoop using any tool, the sequence of events that follows is explained below:

- Client submits the job to the JobTracker which is a component of Hadoop. JobTracker is a point of failure for Hadoop. If the JobTracker stops working, the entire setup fails.

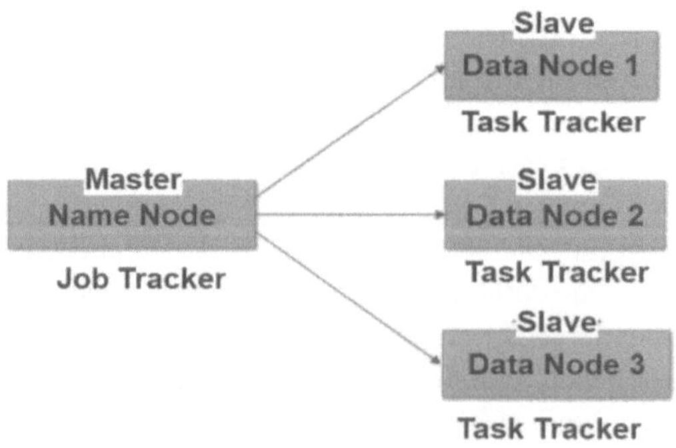

FIGURE 8.3 Master slave architecture.

- The JobTracker polls the Name Node to find which Data Nodes contain the required data. Since the Name Node contains data about the entire file system, it is another point of failure.
- Then the JobTracker will submit the tasks to the respective TaskTrackers.
- The TaskTracker constantly informs the JobTracker that it is alive via heartbeats. If the TaskTracker fails to send its heartbeat, this means that it has failed. In such a scenario, JobTracker looks for another Name Node that can complete its task.
- The TaskTracker submits the data to the JobTracker.
- The Client constantly polls the JobTracker for information. When the JobTracker gets the information from TaskTracker, the Client is automatically informed.

In 2003, Hadoop began with a single tool MapReduce containing a simple storage system. However, with time, Hadoop has accumulated a large plethora of software and technologies making it one of the most famous platforms for processing Big Data. Emergence of Big Data [7] in market was proposed by authors where need of tools required to handle these big data sets was required. In another research, authors proposed an architecture [14] which uses tree (i.e., FB+) that forms fast indexing structure using multi-level Key ranges (similar to B+ trees). Range and its point searches are done on the basis of early termination of searches for non-existent data. Next [21], the authors discussed the awareness of privacy integrity and security and discussed issues related to the definition of framework which supports the access control features into existing Big Data platforms.

8.2.3 Spark

The previous section talked about Hadoop terminology. Often Spark [35] and Hadoop are considered the same with both technologies providing a similar set of functionalities. It is built up of Spark Core and additional libraries. Since Hadoop is based on YARN-based architecture which also enables Spark and other Big Data technologies to share a common cluster and file storage system. Apache Spark is fast and more efficient as compared to previous technologies developed providing streaming data analysis, faster iterative methods to analyse large data sets, and built-in memory engine which supports faster processing of queries over data sets.

It is open source as well. In addition to functionality provided by Hadoop, it also provides SQL query support, graphical data processing, machine learning algorithms, etc. Algorithms which require multi-pass computations are not previously supported by Hadoop and MapReduce systems. With the development of Spark this was made possible, thus gaining an edge over others. It is 100 times faster when executing on memory than previous technologies. Higher level Application Programming Interfaces (APIs) results in optimized performance and also faster performance. Least costly shuffles are provided by Spark as compared to MapReduce. Spark is written in Scala programming language and runs on Java Virtual Machine. As of now, it supports applications to be built in Scala, Java, Python, Clojure and R. Often Spark is thought of as a modified version of Hadoop, but it is wrong to think of it as

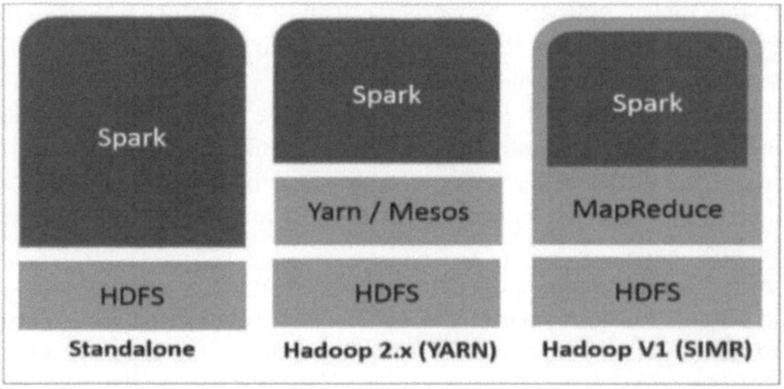

FIGURE 8.4 Implementation of Spark.

such. Using Apache Spark, an application was proposed [5] where a Location-Aware Analytics System was built using spatio-textual indexes and incremental algorithms accepted widely. In [27], the authors proposed a new method for gathering and analysing Twitter data, supported by a larger set of methodological which began to address some of its limitations.

Figure 8.4 shows the three ways through which Spark can be built with Hadoop components. In Standalone mode, Spark and MapReduce run parallelly, with common Hadoop File System and individual results. In Hadoop YARN mode, Spark runs on YARN cluster without any prior installation. In SIMR, i.e., Spark in MapReduce mode, Spark can be used in addition to Standalone mode.

In Figure 8.5, the components [36] of Spark (i.e., Spark SQL, Spark Core, GraphX, Spark Streaming, and Machine Learning Library (MLib)) are discussed: Spark SQL provides SQL support to users where they can write and submit queries to be operated upon data. It is due to Spark Streaming component that real time streaming analysis is made possible. Spark Core consists of the execution engine on which all other components are built. MLib extends the power of Spark by providing machine learning support in Spark where users can design and train machine learning models accordingly. Pregel Abstraction API provides graphical support to users.

Figure 8.6 shows the iterative operations on Spark Resilient Distributed Datasets (RDDs). Immediate results are stored in distributed memory instead of disk.

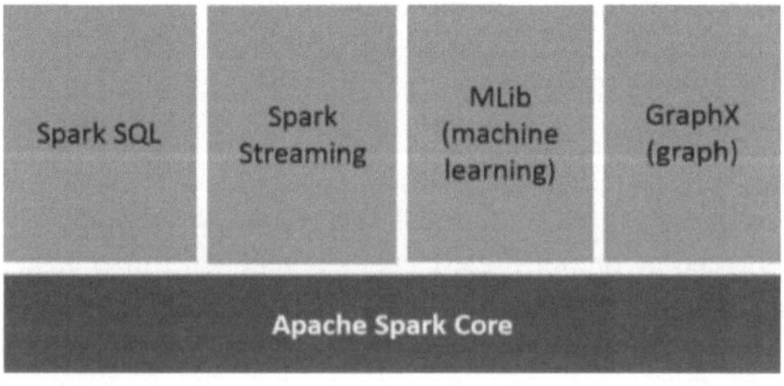

FIGURE 8.5 Components of Spark.

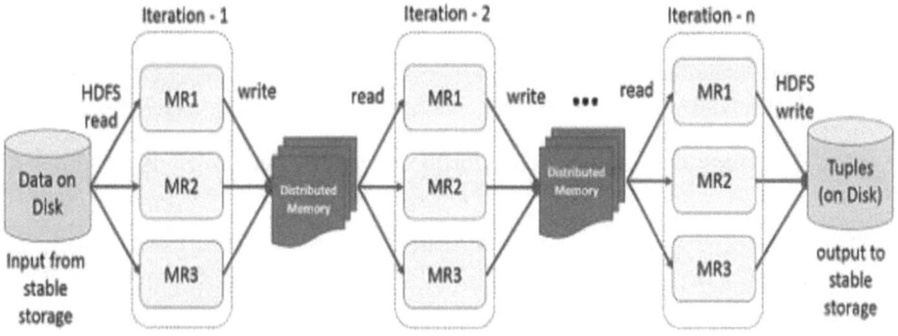

FIGURE 8.6 Iterative operations on Spark.

In-memory computation is the strength of Spark. Disk input/output (I/O), replication, etc. were slow in MapReduce programming. Therefore, the RDD approach was used in Spark. Data sharing is more than 50 times faster as compared to MapReduce.

Figure 8.7 shows the interactive operations on RDD. Data put inside the memory of multiple queries are required to be executed again and again on the same data set. This results in faster performance and increased efficiency. Data is often replicated on multiple nodes, as well to cope with any failure. Spark can be installed on the Ubuntu system using the following procedure:

- Verify that Java is installed using command:
  `java -version`
- Ensure that Hadoop is successfully installed on machine using command:
  `Jps`
- Download Spark form Apache sites and extract these files to execute:
- Edit bashrc:
  Command: `sudo gedit. bashrc`
  Path needs to be set by adding these lines:
  `export SPARK _ HOME=/usr/local/spark`
  `export PATH=$SPARK _ HOME/bin:$PATH`

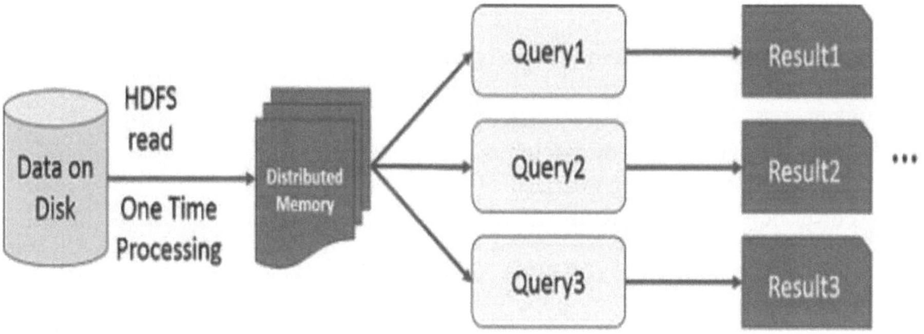

FIGURE 8.7 Interactive operations on Spark.

- Execute bashrc:
  Command: `vi. ~/.bashrc`
- Test the installation:
  Command: `spark-shell`

A basic ETL (Extract, Load and Transform) task can be performed using following process:

- Start Spark's scala-shell:
  Command: `spark-shell`
- Load the file from local file system:
```
scala> var Data = sc.textFile("/user/spark/CHANGES.txt")
//file can be loaded from HDFS as well
```
- Split each line:
```
scala> var tokens = Data.flatMap(s => s.split(" "))
```
- Append 1 with each individual word:
```
scala> var tokens _ 1 = tokens.map(s => (s,1))
```
- Calculate the occurrence of each individual word:
```
scala> var sum _ each = tokens _ 1.reduceByKey((a, b) => a + b)
```
- Save output to a file in local file system:
```
sum _ each.saveAsTextFile("/user/spark _ out")
```
- Examine the ouput

Various other operations can be performed as well using Spark. Python can be used as well instead of Scala in Spark's Python PySpark Shell. An application on deep learning and Spark was proposed in this research as well [37].

Advantages of Spark

- Cluster computing
- Supports GraphX, MLib, and other components
- Provides real-time streaming data analysis
- Flexible and powerful
- Uses same platform for both real-time and batch processing

Disadvantages of Spark

- Consumes a larger memory space
- Takes a large amount of resources
- No File Management System of its own
- Fewer number of algorithms in MLib

8.2.4 Pig

Pig works over MapReduce as a higher level of abstraction that was originated by Yahoo in 2006 and it moved into the Foundation of the Apache Software in 2007.

It has some unique characteristics which make it good in processing a large amount of data. There are often various challenges that we need to face while handling this amount of data.

In [3], the authors give different methods to tackle challenges like computational, system, and data complexity; whereas, challenges of visual analytics and exemplifying them with several applications and their limitations [32] are discussed as follows:

- Pig Latin [38] uses simple language for writing code to process data.
- Its code is internally converted into MapReduce due to its high level of abstract nature.
- Users can define their own function which can be written like other programming languages such as, Java, etc.
- While comparing with MapReduce, it needed a smaller amount of code.
- Users have two mode of execution, i.e., local and MapReduce modes.
- Pig has functionality to use a multiple-query approach, which helps to minimize the size of code.
- Pig Engine helps to optimize the code. The tasks in Pig are automatically optimized by the Pig Engine.

Pig can be installed on the Ubuntu system using the following procedure:

- Verify if Hadoop is installed; Command: `jps`
- If it is not installed, then download from Apache site and unzip that file to further execute. To check the version of Pig, type command: `pig-version`.

After installation, Pig is successfully set up (as shown in Figure 8.8), Pig commands can be executed inside Grunt Shell, and output is stored in Pig order result directory on HDFS.

However, the main advantage of Pig is that it handles three different types of data (i.e., Structured, Semi-structured, and Unstructured) easily using the same tools.

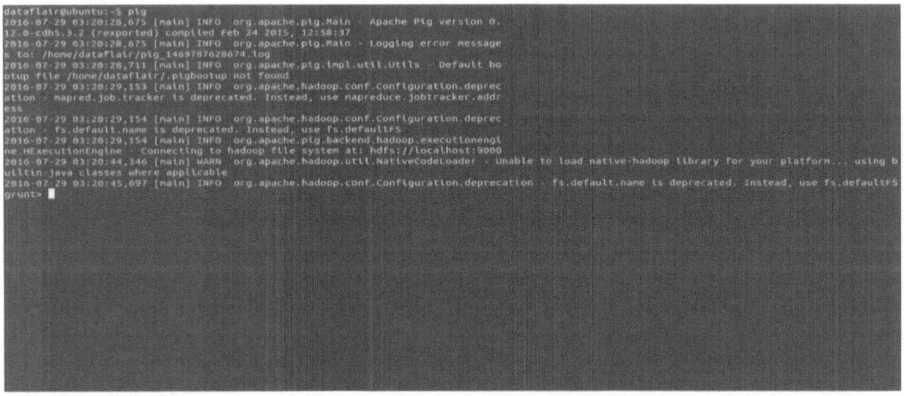

FIGURE 8.8 Pig installed.

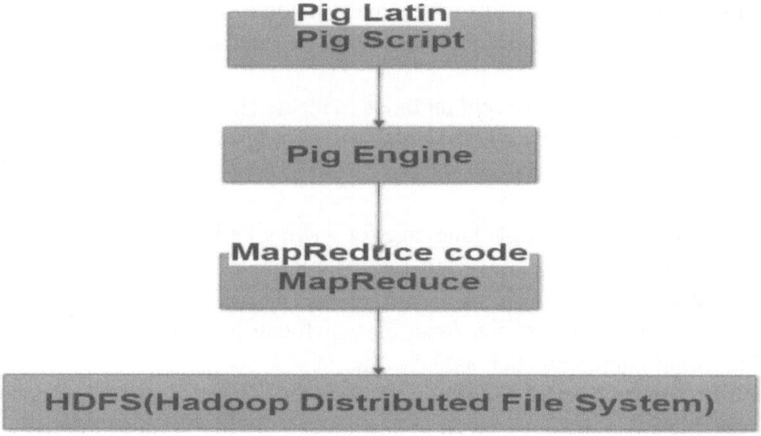

FIGURE 8.9 Pig architecture.

Compilation and execution phases are described in detail in one research [39]. It defined Pig into parts: Latin Pig and Pig Engine, as shown in Figure 8.9. Latin Pig (i.e., high level language) is used to write all the Pig scripts; whereas, Pig Engine is the execution engine that takes Pig script as input and produces output in the form of MapReduce code. The generated code runs on Hadoop platform (i.e., HDFS) and produces the information. Parser, Grunt Shell, Optimizer, Pig server, execution engine, and compiler are the various parts of Pig Engine.

In conclusion, even Pig needs to convert the input code into MapReduce code which is a time-consuming process, even though Pig has been used by many due to its simplicity and ease to learn.

8.2.5 MapReduce

MapReduce is defined as a software framework which is used to build applications and programs to process large amounts of data parallelly on multiple machines. As the name suggests, it consists of two major phases: Map and Reduce [42] in addition to the Splitting phase

The Map phase considers raw data as an input and produces an intermediate data set consisting of key/value pairs. The Reduce phase takes the intermediate data set from all the mappers as input and produces a single set of key/value pairs as output. The Reduce step can itself be partitioned into three different phases, namely Shuffle phase, Sort phase and Reduce phase. All these phases have been discussed in detail with an example. It is basically a programming model for processing large data sets. In [8], the authors proposed a model which takes Map and Reduce functions to parallelize the computation (automatically) across large-scale clusters of machines. It also helps to handle failures of machines, and schedules communication between inter-machine to efficiently utilize the network and disks.

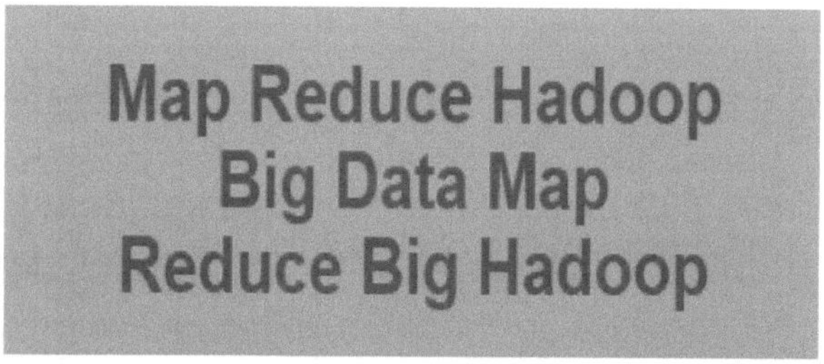

FIGURE 8.10 Input data.

A working structure of MapReduce is shown in Figure 8.10. The three phases are summarized below:

- **Splitting Phase:** The raw data is split into different chunks of data as shown in Figure 8.11. The number of splits is equivalent to the number of mappers available since each chunk of data is sent to one mapper.
- **Map Phase:** This phase takes the input chunk of data from the HDFS and converts it into an Intermediate Dataset as shown in Figure 8.12. The Intermediate Dataset consists of tuples (key/value) of data. The tasks that convert raw data into intermediate data are called Maps.
- **Reduce Phase:** The Reduce phase is further divided into three sub-phases as shown in Figure 8.13:
  - **Shuffle phase** by which the Intermediate Dataset is transferred from mappers to one or multiple Reducers.
  - **Sort phase** in which the Reducer groups the input by keys.
  - **Reduce phase** in which the Reducer processes the intermediate data received from the Mappers and produces the final output. The number of Reducers used is equivalent to the number of outputs required.

Other facilities available in MapReduce are the following:

- **Reporter:** It is used to report the progress of the MapReduce task. The Mapper and Reducer can use the Reporter to report their progress. Further, it can also be used by these programs as an indication that they are alive and

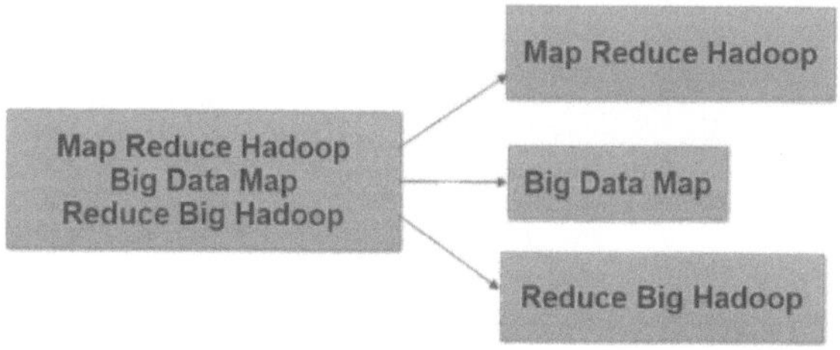

FIGURE 8.11 Splitting phase.

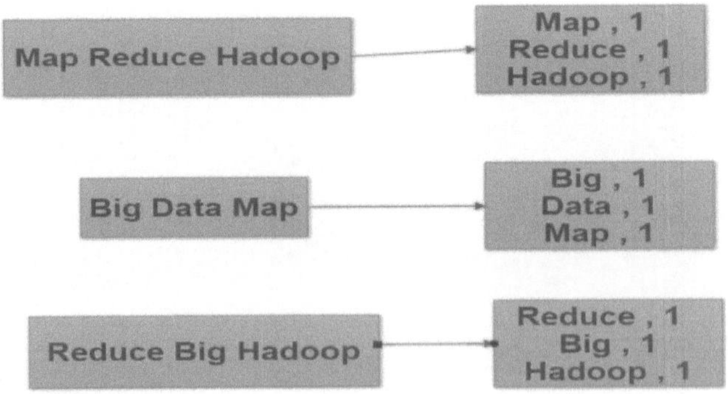

FIGURE 8.12 Map phase.

working. This becomes necessary when the program is consuming a lot of time and the framework is about to kill it.

- **Output Collector:** It is used to collect the output from Mappers and Reducers.

The authors [10] characterized the MapReduce framework and discussed its pros and cons. Also, the optimization strategies reported in the recent literature as well as open issues and challenges raised on parallel data analysis with MapReduce are discussed. Further, they analysed several potential strategies (i.e., data analytics placement) along with I/O path and chose the best strategy to overcome the data movement in a given situation. Flex Analytics system works over HEC platform to improve the scalability and flexibility of current I/O stack which is useful for runtime data analysis, data pre-processing for transfer of data at a large scale [23]. A sample implementation of Financial Analysis of Goldman Sachs Stock Data is shown in Table 8.1.

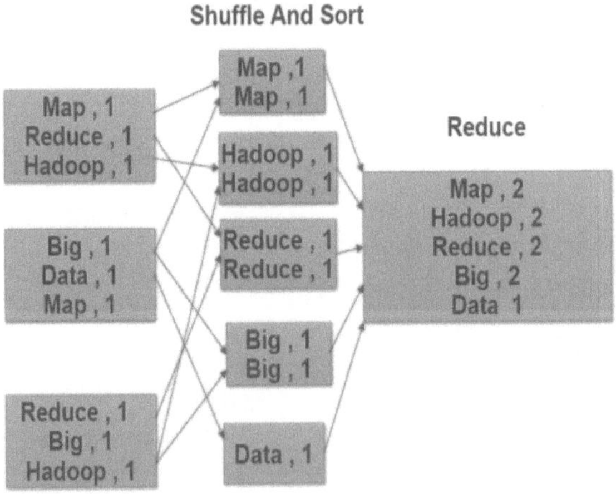

FIGURE 8.13 Reduce phase.

TABLE 8.1
Sample Data

Date	Open	High	Low	Last	Close	Total Trade Quantity	Turnover (Lacs)	Id
2019-08-26	2836	2854.7	2825.4	2843	2841.55	8264	234.81	1
2019-08-25	2835	2839.85	2825.5	2833.9	2831.75	5958	168.87	2
2019-08-24	2848.1	2855	2842.6	2853.5	2852	4472	127.41	3
2019-08-23	2855	2863.8	2845.1	2845.4	2848.45	6615	188.78	4

Full data is stored in sampledata.txt in HDFS.

- A new directory is created
  Command: `mkdir sample`
- File is moved from local file system to HDFS
  Command: `$HADOOP _ HOME/bin/hadoop fs -put/home/hadoop/sampledata.txt input _ dir`

Benefits of Using MapReduce

- **Parallel Computing:** MapReduce distributes the task amongst various systems. This is known as parallel computing which distributes the load among various systems and improves the performance of the overall system.
- **Scalability:** Since the data is divided amongst multiple systems, it is capable of dealing with large amounts of data by increasing the number of nodes.
- **Low Cost:** MapReduce does not require costly computers to process data. The jobs are executed on commodity hardware. Hence, the total cost of processing MapReduce jobs is less.
- **Faster Time:** Since the task is conducted simultaneously on multiple nodes, the total time required to complete a task is less than using other technologies.
- **Recovery:** When the data is stored on HDFS, the framework stores data simultaneously in multiple locations. Hence, in the scenario of a system crash and subsequent loss of data, data can be recovered from the remaining locations.
- **Simple:** The users are not required to learn an additional language to process data using MapReduce. Languages like Java and Python can be used to write MapReduce code.
- **Locality of Reference:** The Job Tracker and Name Node are responsible for assigning tasks to the nodes. These attempt to assign the tasks to the nodes that have data on the local disk. Hence, there is minimal movement of data from node to node.

New MapReduce research trends were proposed in a study [11] in which the authors concluded that the direction of research in MapReduce concerned either enhancing its programming model or deploying existing algorithm to run on this model.

Disadvantages of Using MapReduce

- MapReduce is designed for Online Analytical Processing (OLAP) systems only. It cannot be used in Online Transaction Processing (OLTP) systems.
- Since MapReduce processes the data on multiple systems simultaneously, the entire system needs to be set up prior to processing data.
- The MapReduce code is written in Java or Python. Hence, working knowledge of one of these languages is a must for MapReduce.
- It is only useful in applications where the task can be divided amongst multiple nodes.

An application [30] was proposed based on MapReduce where image file e-books are converted into text file e-books to enable searching for words in e-books.

8.2.6 Kafka

Most of the technologies that were developed before the introduction of Kafka handled unstreamed and static data. There existed technologies that worked upon streaming data [41], but their efficiency and performance was not up to the mark as required with the current technology advancements. Also, not all data is fit to be streamed, but trends are shifting towards streaming data analysis. Today one-third of the Fortune 500 Companies use Kafka whether they are from the telecom, travel, and banking sectors, and much more. Kafka has laid its roots everywhere with its real-time analytics supported by powerful architecture of HDFS which is a distributed file system that allows storing of static data, and hence batch processing can be done on a database. This type of architecture provides analysis where results on historical data or any past data is required. But this approach fails where processing of future messages is required as well. This does not mean Kafka cannot process past data, instead what it does is it goes up to the last record stored in the database and keeps on processing the future data upon arrival. Therefore, it is an extension to previously designed technologies thus providing extensive functionality over them. Originally developed at LinkedIn, Kafka steadily made its presence felt in markets among various enterprises.

Using Apache Kafka [4], the authors proposed a system for forecasting of electricity generation that can predict the required power generation (i.e., close to 99% of the actual usage) by using Big Data Analytics. It is often compared to other technologies like ActiveMQ or RabbitMQ for implementation in enterprises, but with its ability to handle high velocity data streams, other technologies fade away. Since being developed at LinkedIn, it has a high-profile support from big companies like Netflix, Uber and others. It was written in Scala and Java originally by its developers. It has a built-in partitioning system, offers high throughput, better fault-tolerance system in case system failure occurs and a great large-scale messaging system. It can be integrated with Apache Spark and Apache Storm for real-time analysis. Log aggregation solution is another area where Kafka is useful. It collects logs from various services across organizations and makes them available in required format for consumers. In Kafka, data is stored in the form of topics which is nothing but a stream of messages which belong together. These topics are broken down into partitions, and each partition contains a subset of the original topic. Creation of partitions eases out the processing, and a larger amount of data can be handled using this approach. Kafka architecture has four core APIs:

- **Producer API:** Producers are the publishers which send data to Kafka brokers. Whenever a producer sends a message to a broker, then the brokers simply appends the data at the end of the partition. Producer has a choice between either to send data to partition of its own choice or broker append to the last partition or any default one.
- **Consumer API:** Consumers consume data from brokers or in simple words they access the data from brokers. They subscribe the topics according to their requirements and pull the data from brokers for further processing. Data can be easily accessed in Kafka cluster due to its policy of partition creation.
- **Stream API:** Stream API takes input from various topics, processes them and generates outputs to be presented to one or more topics. These APIs are useful if data items need to be accessed from one topic to another.
- **Connector API:** Connector APIs connect the topics to applications. Also, they identify the reusable producers and consumers which can link the topics with applications. These APIs are necessary from both the user as well as system point of view.

Because of its rich set of features, various companies hire Kafka experts. The salary trends for this domain have increased significantly over the years providing more and more opportunities in this sector as well. Figure 8.14 shows the cluster diagram of a Kafka ecosystem.

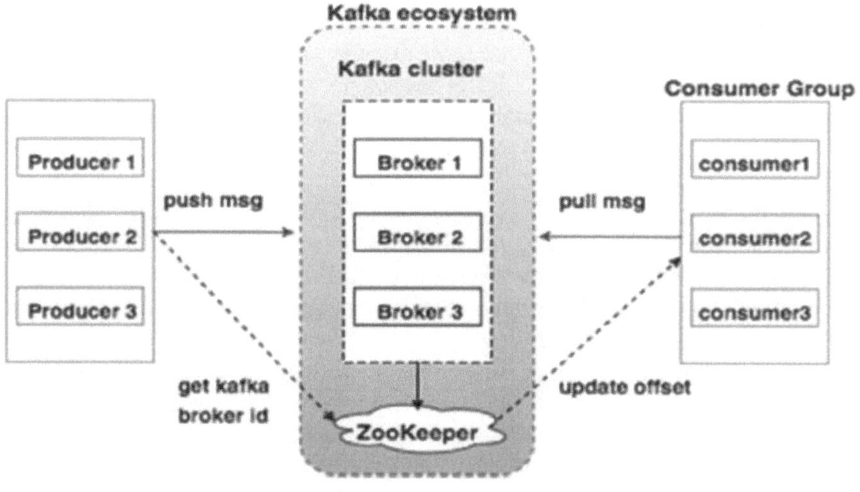

FIGURE 8.14 Kafka ecosystem [40].

There are four major components shown in this diagram:

- **Brokers:** These are the load balancers of a Kafka cluster. There are multiple brokers inside a cluster to handle large amounts of data. Each broker can handle thousands of reads and writes per second which in turn contain terabytes of messages without any impact on performance. They are stateless and a leader is selected among all the brokers by ZooKeeper.
- **ZooKeepers:** These are the managers of all the brokers present in the system. They provide information to producers and consumers if any new broker is added in the system or when there is failure of any present broker. All the broker activities are coordinated by ZooKeeper. Depending upon the information provided by ZooKeeper to consumers and producers, necessary action is taken by them, i.e., whether to work with a new broker or any other thing.
- **Producers:** As the data arrives to a Kafka cluster, producers seamlessly push the data to brokers irrespective of any acknowledgement. New data is appended at the end of brokers. From there on, processing of data takes place.
- **Consumers:** Data stored inside brokers are used by consumers. They issue pull requests as opposed to push requests made by producers. Every partition has an offset value attached with itself. An asynchronous request is made depicting how many bytes of data it has to consume according to requirement. ZooKeeper also plays an important role here of notifying the consumer offset value. It totally depends on the consumer how many topics it has to subscribe, which message to be skipped, which to be escaped and many more.

Offset values of a message are maintained by ZooKeeper. Once the producer pushes the data into cluster, an offset value is assigned to every message by ZooKeeper. The Consumer issues the pull request to ZooKeeper, accesses the data, processes it and sends an acknowledgement back to ZooKeeper after completion of task. Upon receiving the acknowledgement, the offset values of the accessed messages are updated with the new values. ZooKeeper can be thought of as a synchronization mechanism between consumers and brokers to provide smooth functionality across the system. In case of system failure, a new leader among all the brokers needs to be selected which is done by the ZooKeeper. Also from time to time, the ZooKeeper replicates the data stored inside Kafka brokers to handle the system failure situation which in turn is one of the major strengths of Kafka. Kafka can be set up in two configurations again depending upon requirements. One is a single broker cluster and the other is a multi-broker cluster.

Figure 8.15 shows the setup of Apache Kafka with single node-single broker and single ZooKeeper configuration. There are multiple producers and consumers present in the system. Figure 8.16 shows an overview of a Kafka system with single node-multiple brokers and single ZooKeeper configuration. Here also there are multiple producers and consumers. Four major benefits of Kafka are Scalability, Reliability, Durability, and Performance.

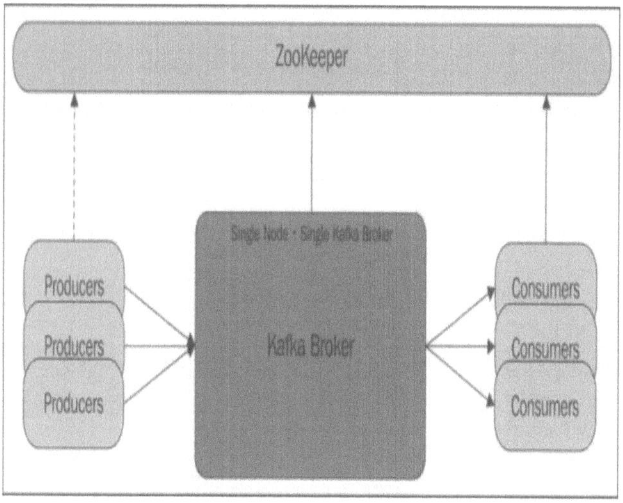

FIGURE 8.15 Single node-single broker [40].

Kafka can be installed using the following process:

- Verify Java Installation
- ZooKeeper Framework is installed
  i. Download ZooKeeper
  ii. Extract tar file
  iii. Create Configuration File
  iv. Start ZooKeeper Server
  v. Start CLI

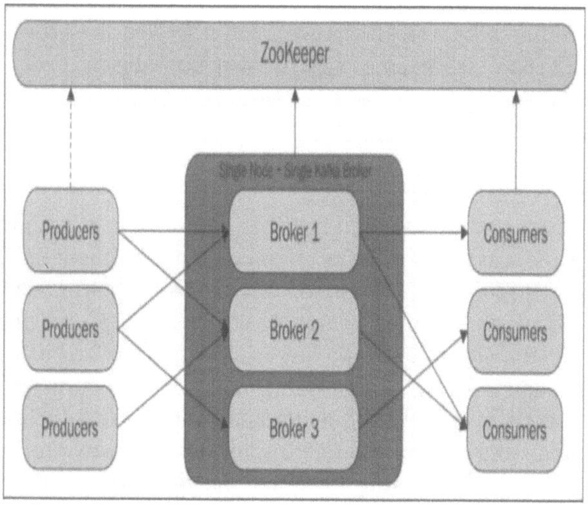

FIGURE 8.16 Single node-multiple broker [40].

- Apache Kafka is installed
  1. Download Kafka
  2. Extract tar file
  3. Start Kafka Server

After installation of ZooKeeper and Kafka, single node-single broker can be implemented using the following steps:

- Start ZooKeeper
- Configure Single Node-Single Broker
  i. Get List of Topics
    Command: `bin/kafka-topics.sh -list -zookeeper localhost:2181`
  ii. Send Message
    Command: `bin/kafka-console-producer.sh -broker-list localhost:9092 -topic topic-name`
  iii. Receive Message
    Command: `bin/kafka-console-consumer.sh -zoo-keeper localhost:2181 –topic topic-name` –from-beginning
- Single Node-Multiple Broker system can be configured similarly
- Some topic operations:
  1. Modify Topic
    Command: `bin/kafka-topics.sh –zookeeper local-host:2181 -alter -topic topic _ name -parti-tions count`
    Example: `bin/kafka-topics.sh -zookeeper localhost:2181 -alter -topic Hello-kafka -parti-tions 2`
  2. Delete Topic
    Command: `bin/kafka-topics.sh -zookeeper local-host:2181 -delete -topic topic _ name`
    Example: `bin/kafka-topics.sh -zookeeper local-host:2181 -delete -topic Hello-kafka`

User can interact with Kafka by writing interactive queries and generating results thereby. This system analysed several possible data-analytics assignment strategies with an I/O path and was quite able to overcome data movement in a given situation.

A Flex Analytics [24] system improves the flexibility and scalability of present I/O stack on HEC platforms and is valuable for data pre-processing, runtime data analysis as well as transfer of data at a large scale. Kafka can be downloaded from kafka.apache.org, and its setup generally includes some moderate prerequisites like Java which should be installed in systems and others. With the current advancements in technology and enterprises looking for best systems in the market, Kafka has proved its presence from time to time. The overview of Kafka is shown in Figure 8.17.

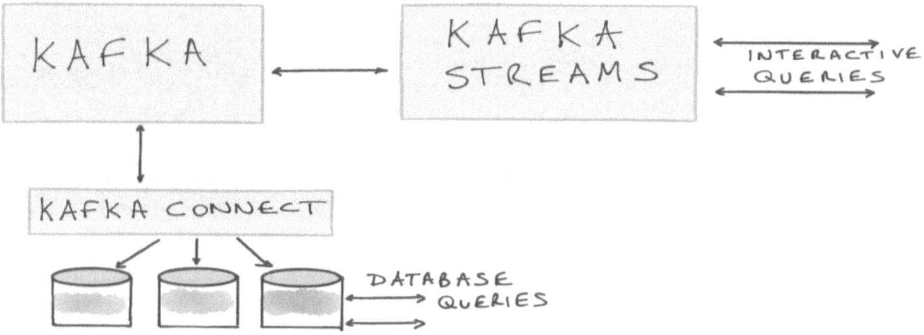

FIGURE 8.17 Kafka overview [24].

8.2.7 Hive

Hive is used in Hadoop as a data warehouse infrastructure which processes structured data. It exists on top of Hadoop to digest Big Data, and makes querying and analyzing easy. Facebook (a company) was the one that developed Hive at the initial stage; later, the Apache Software Foundation took it up, declared it as an open source, and named it Apache Hive. A detailed study was discussed in [34] on Hive and HiveQL. Hive was designed for Online Analytical Processing (OLAP). It stores schema in a database as an SQL type query (i.e., HiveQL, or HQL) and processed data into HDFC. Hive's features are fast, scalable, familiar, and extensible.

The working of Hive is as follows:

- **Execute Query:** It consists of Hive interface such as Command Line or maybe Web UI for sending query to Driver (any database driver such as JDBC, ODBC, etc.) for execution.
- **Get Metadata:** The compiler transmits metadata request to any Metastore (database).
- **Get Plan:** The driver takes advantage of the query compiler that parses the same query to check the query's syntax, plan and requirement.
- **Send Plan:** Further, the compiler checks the requirement then retransmits the plan to the driver for completing and parsing the query.
- **Send Metadata:** It is responsible to transmit metadata as a response to the compiler.
- **Execute Plan:** The driver transmits the execute plan to the execution engine.
- **Metadata Ops:** During execution, the execution engine executes metadata operations with Metastore.
- **Execute Job:** Internally, the execution job process is a MapReduce job. The execution engine transmits the job to JobTracker, which is in Name Node and it assigns this.
- **Fetch and send Result:** The execution engine receives the results from Data Nodes. The execution engine sends those resultant values to the driver; the driver sends the results to Hive Interfaces.

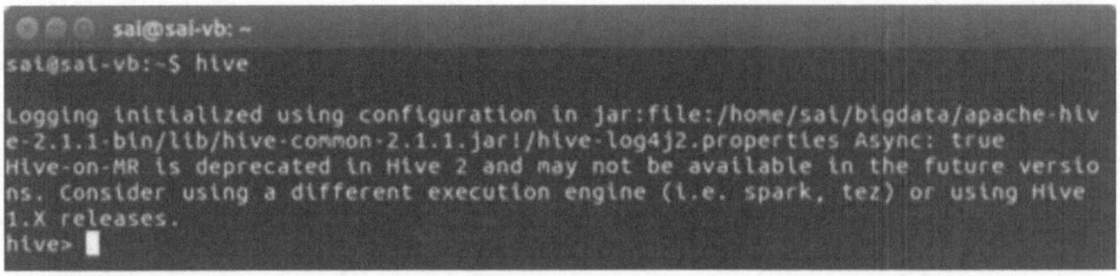

FIGURE 8.18 Hive installed.

Hive can be installed using the following steps:

- Verify Hadoop installation.
  Command: `jps`
- If it is not installed, then download its tar file, extract it and configure it.
- Initialize Derby database
- Launch Hive

Now that Hive is successfully set up as shown in Figure 8.18, Hive commands can be executed. Output generated from the query could be stored on HDFS in USER directory.

Advantages of Hive

- Higher level query language
- Less trial-and-error than Pig
- Support of external tables
- Partitioning of data is possible
- Built on top of Hadoop

Disadvantages of Hive

- Real-time processing is not possible
- High latency
- Comparatively slow
- Updating and modification is difficult

8.3 BIG DATA IN E-HEALTHCARE

As we discussed in Section 8.2 about the working structure of Big Data and its functionality, Big Data works wonders for a massive amount of data. Many organizations (either public or private) focus on storing, analysing and generating Big Data with the aim to improve their services provided to the users (or customers). Healthcare industries are more concerned with managing patient data and diagnosing their patients after analysis of these collected data. Healthcare is a multi-disciplinary system that aims to diagnose disease and prevent human beings from having a disease. The main components of a healthcare system are doctors, nurses, pharmacies, clinics, hospitals, etc. Healthcare is required with many types of urgency. A professional

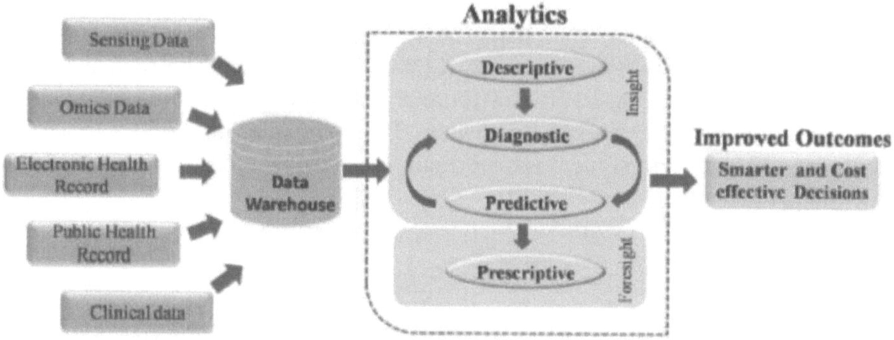

FIGURE 8.19 Big Data in healthcare [44].

cures a patients by knowing their past medical history. In the old times, a patient's medical record was written in a note pad or in any type of report. Even the patient examination result was stored in a file system (i.e., in paper form). In the present time, these records are maintained in the form of a log file or in any electronic way. These methods keep patients' health records, but as time passes, this data becomes massive and handling of this huge amount of data is a difficult task. Then healthcare industries move to Big Data which is quite able to handle huge amounts of data with the concept of a data warehouse. Electronic Health Record (EHR) and Electronic Medical Record (EMR), among others, are collectively improving the health record data which ultimately improves people's health-related issues. Figure 8.19 shows the role of Big Data in healthcare includes the healthcare payer-provider data (such as EMRs, pharmacy prescription, and insurance records) along with the genomics-driven experiments (such as genotyping, gene expression data) and other data acquired from the smart Web of the Internet of Things (IoT) [44].

8.4 CONCLUSION

Many mobile applications or biometric sensors generate a large amount of data related to healthcare. This is very important to understand generated data and overcome issues of this generated data by different health-monitoring applications. In this chapter, we have discussed the most used technologies for handling Big Data starting from the old-school methods of manual analysis and moving on to advanced technologies like Spark, Kafka, etc. Some of these technologies like manual analysis and MRP systems have been replaced by new technologies. However, a plethora of technologies still exist in the market. As a result, organizations dealing with Big Data have to choose the right technology to use for handling Big Data related to the healthcare industry. The main question that arises when choosing the correct platform is what the requirements of the organization are and what outcome they expect if they deploy a certain scheme. In addition, the managers have to take cost and storage factors into account as well. Selecting the right platform is a tough as well as a complicated step. Furthermore, once an organization commits, then adopting something different is difficult as well as expensive. Every major company and organization is using Big Data in today's time to organize large amounts of health-related data. The use of Big Data has grown to encompass multiple industries and fields. Big Data facilitates healthcare in terms of predicting health-related issues. After analysis of Big Data, EHRs, EMRs and other medical data are continuously helping build a better prognostic framework. The companies providing service for healthcare analytics and clinical transformation are indeed contributing towards a better and effective outcome.

REFERENCES

[1] Sakr, S. and Elgammal, A., 2016. Towards a comprehensive data analytics framework for smart healthcare services. *Big Data Research*, *4*, pp. 44–58.
[2] Chen, Z., Xu, G., Mahalingam, V., Ge, L., Nguyen, J., Yu, W. and Lu, C., 2016. A cloud computing based network monitoring and threat detection system for critical infrastructures. *Big Data Research*, *3*, pp. 10–23.
[3] Jin, X., Wah, B.W., Cheng, X. and Wang, Y., 2015. Significance and challenges of big data research. *Big Data Research*, *2*(2), pp. 59–64.
[4] Rahman, M.N., Esmailpour, A. and Zhao, J., 2016. Machine learning with big data an efficient electricity generation forecasting system. *Big Data Research*, *5*, pp. 9–15.
[5] Liu, Y., Wang, H., Li, G., Gao, J., Hu, H. and Li, W.S., 2016. ELAN: An efficient location-aware analytics system. *Big Data Research*, *5*, pp. 16–21.
[6] Chaudhuri, S., 2012, May. What next? A half-dozen data management research goals for big data and the cloud. In Proceedings of the 31st ACM SIGMOD-SIGACT-SIGAI symposium on Principles of Database Systems (pp. 1–4).
[7] Nunan, D. and Di Domenico, M., 2013. Market research and the ethics of big data. *International Journal of Market Research*, *55*(4), pp. 505–520.
[8] Dean, J. and Ghemawat, S., 2004. MapReduce: Simplified data processing on large clusters. In OSDI '04: 6th Symposium on Operating Systems Design and Implementation, USENIX Association.
[9] Dean, J. and Ghemawat, S., 2008. MapReduce: simplified data processing on large clusters. *Communications of the ACM*, *51*(1), pp. 107–113.
[10] Lee, K.H., Lee, Y.J., Choi, H., Chung, Y.D. and Moon, B., 2012. Parallel data processing with MapReduce: a survey. *AcM sIGMoD Record*, *40*(4), pp. 11–20.
[11] Abdelrahman Elsayed, O.I. and El-Sharkawi, M.E., 2014. MapReduce: State-of-the-art and research directions. *International Journal of Computer and Electrical Engineering*, *6*(1).
[12] Wu, X., Zhu, X., Wu, G.Q. and Ding, W., 2013. Data mining with big data. *IEEE Transactions on Knowledge and Data Engineering*, *26*(1), pp. 97–107.
[13] De Gennaro, M., Paffumi, E. and Martini, G., 2016. Big data for supporting low-carbon road transport policies in Europe: Applications, challenges and opportunities. *Big Data Research*, *6*, pp. 11–25.
[14] Yu, C. and Boyd, J., 2016. FB+-tree for big data management. *Big Data Research*, *4*, pp. 25–36.
[15] Diamantoulakis, P.D., Kapinas, V.M. and Karagiannidis, G.K., 2015. Big data analytics for dynamic energy management in smart grids. *Big Data Research*, *2*(3), pp. 94–101.
[16] Pääkkönen, P. and Pakkala, D., 2015. Reference architecture and classification of technologies, products and services for big data systems. *Big Data Research*, *2*(4), pp. 166–186.
[17] Seo, Y. and Ahn, J., 2013. User taste prediction service using big data. *Advanced Science and Technology Letters*, 29, pp. 295–298. D.O.I: 10.14257/astl.2013.29.62.

[18] Hong, B.H. and Joo, H.J., 2013. A study on the Monitoring Model for Traffic Analysis and Application of Big Data. *International research on Big Data, Seoul, Korea*, 43, pp. 30–35.
[19] Dagli, M.K. and Mehta, B.B., 2014. Big data and Hadoop: a review. *International Journal of Applied Research in Engineering and Science*, *2*(2), p. 192.
[20] Ang, L.M. and Seng, K.P., 2016. Big sensor data applications in urban environments. *Big Data Research*, *4*, pp. 1–12.
[21] Rahman, M.N. and Esmailpour, A., 2016. A hybrid data center architecture for big data. *Big Data Research*, *3*, pp. 29–40.
[22] Colombo, P. and Ferrari, E., 2015. Privacy aware access control for big data: A research roadmap. *Big Data Research*, *2*(4), pp. 145–154.
[23] Kolomvatsos, K., Anagnostopoulos, C. and Hadjiefthymiades, S., 2015. An efficient time optimized scheme for progressive analytics in big data. *Big Data Research*, *2*(4), pp. 155–165.
[24] Zou, H., Yu, Y., Tang, W. and Chen, H.W.M., 2014. FlexAnalytics: a flexible data analytics framework for big data applications with I/O performance improvement. *Big Data Research*, *1*, pp. 4–13.
[25] Schenker, N., 2013. Big-Data: Uses and Limitations. Paper presented at the National Center for Health Statistics Centers for Disease Control and Prevention.
[26] Brauer, E.K., Singh, D.K. and Popescu, S.C., 2014. Next-generation plant science: putting big data to work. *Genome Biology, 15:301.*
[27] Tinati, R., Halford, S., Carr, L. and Pope, C., 2013. The promise of big data: new methods for sociological analysis. *The World Social Science Forum, 7 pp.*
[28] Leavitt, N., 2013. Storage challenge: Where will all that big data go?. *Computer*, (9), pp. 22–25.
[29] Ferguson, D. and Catterson, V., 2014. Big data techniques for wind turbine condition monitoring. Paper presented at the *European Wind Energy Association Annual Event (EWEA 2014), Barcelona, Spain.*
[30] Hong, T.H., Yun, C.H., Park, J.W., Lee, H.G., Jung, H.S. and Lee, Y.W., 2013. Big data processing with MapReduce for E-book. *International Journal of Multimedia and Ubiquitous Engineering*, *8*(1), pp. 151–162.
[31] Lee, C.W., Cho, S.H., Kim, J.W. and Hwang, D.H., 2013. A study on improvements of electric trading system using big data. *Advanced Science and Technology Letters*, 43, pp. 114–118.
[32] Keim, D., 2013. Solving problems with visual analytics: The role of visualization and analytics in exploring big data. *Datenbanksysteme für Business, Technologie und Web (BTW) 2013.*
[33] Chirkova, R. and Yang, J., 2013. Big and useful: what's in the data for me?. *Proceedings of the VLDB Endowment*, *6*(12), pp. 1390–1391.
[34] Thusoo, A., Sarma, J.S., Jain, N., Shao, Z., Chakka, P., Zhang, N., Antony, S., Liu, H. and Murthy, R., 2010, March. Hive-a petabyte scale data warehouse using Hadoop. In 2010 IEEE 26th International Conference on Data Engineering (ICDE 2010) (pp. 996–1005). IEEE.
[35] Zaharia, M., Chowdhury, M., Franklin, M.J., Shenker, S. and Stoica, I., 2010. Spark: Cluster computing with working sets. *HotCloud*, *10*(10-10), p. 95.
[36] Fu, J., Sun, J. and Wang, K., 2016, December. Spark–a big data processing platform for machine learning. In 2016 International Conference on Industrial Informatics-Computing Technology, Intelligent Technology, Industrial Information Integration (ICIICII) (pp. 48–51). IEEE.
[37] Gupta, A., Thakur, H.K., Shrivastava, R., Kumar, P. and Nag, S., 2017, November. A big data analysis framework using apache spark and deep learning. In 2017 IEEE International Conference on Data Mining Workshops (ICDMW) (pp. 9–16). IEEE.

[38] Olston, C., Reed, B., Srivastava, U., Kumar, R. and Tomkins, A., 2008, June. Pig Latin: a not-so-foreign language for data processing. In Proceedings of the 2008 ACM SIGMOD International Conference on Management of Data (pp. 1099–1110).
[39] Gates, A.F., Natkovich, O., Chopra, S., Kamath, P., Narayanamurthy, S.M., Olston, C., Reed, B., Srinivasan, S. and Srivastava, U., 2009. Building a high-level dataflow system on top of Map-Reduce: the Pig experience. *Proceedings of the VLDB Endowment*, *2*(2), pp. 1414–1425.
[40] Kreps, J., Narkhede, N. and Rao, J., 2011, June. Kafka: A distributed messaging system for log processing. In Proceedings of the NetDB (Vol. 11, pp. 1–7).
[41] Garg, N., 2015. *Learning Apache Kafka*. Packt Publishing Ltd.: Birmingham, UK.
[42] Gupta, M. and Singla, N., 2019. Evolution of cloud in big data with Hadoop on docker platform. In *Web Services: Concepts, Methodologies, Tools, and Applications* (pp. 1601–1622). IGI Global.
[43] Gupta, M. and Singla, N., 2019. Learner to advanced: big data journey. *Handbook of IoT and Big Data*, p. 187.
[44] Dash, S., Shakyawar, S.K., Sharma, M. and Kaushik, S., 2019. Big data in healthcare: management, analysis and future prospects. *Journal of Big Data*, *6*(1), p. 54.

Index

A

Activities of Daily Living (ADLs) 9
Adaptive care provisioning 44
Anaerobic study 99, 103
Antennas viii, ix, 64, 66–79
Application Programming Interfaces (APIs) 4, 145
ASK: Amplitude Shift Keying 42
Automation 21, 32
Autonomy 3, 52, 131
Azure (Microsoft) 7, 54

B

Base station 64–66
Big Data ix, x, xi, 5, 6, 20, 52, 137–142, 144, 145, 159–162
Biomedical viii, 39–41, 53, 54, 64, 72, 79
Biometric-based security framework 39
Biosensors 7, 53, 54, 64–65
Biosensors and bio-actuators 64, 65
Blockchain viii, 51–59
Bluetooth 4, 8, 12, 14, 41, 42, 53, 75, 99
Borg scale 90, 98
Broadband and wireless networks 20

C

Channel propagation 64, 66
Clinical epidemiology 23
Clinical trials 52–53, 55, 59
Communication protocols vii, 1–4, 8, 14, 28
Connectivity 3, 4, 8, 12, 53
Conversational agents ix, 111, 112, 115, 116, 121, 123, 125, 127, 128
Counterfeit drugs viii, 56
Cryptocurrency viii, 52, 54, 58
Cybersecurity legislation 32

D

Data-driven medicine 20, 23, 25, 32
Data security and patient privacy 14
Data science
Diagnostic 30, 51, 125
Disruptive Civil Technologies 2
DSSS: Direct Sequence Spread Spectrum 42

E

Electroencephalogram (EEG) sensors 10
e-Healthcare ix, 137, 160
Electrocardiogram (ECG) 7, 10
Electronics circuitry 64
Embodied Conversational Agents (ECAs) 112, 115

F

Fake medications viii, 55
Fatigue estimation 83, 85, 92
FHSS: Frequency Hopping Spread Spectrum 42
Functional Magnetic Resonance Imaging (fMRI) 26

G

Graphical User Interfaces (GUIs) 4, 8

H

Hadoop x, 138, 140, 141, 143–146, 153, 159, 160
Health monitoring x, 44, 45, 161
Healthcare delivery ix, 111–115, 117, 129
Healthcare industry x, 2, 9, 22, 161
Heterogeneity 3, 24
Histogram equalization 26

I

IEEE 802.11 – WiFi 8
IEEE 802.15.1 – Bluetooth 8
IEEE 802.16 – WiMAX 8
Image processing 20, 28
Implantable antenna 69, 70, 72
Implantable/sensing antennas 64
Inertial sensors 89, 93
Insulations 64, 65
Internet of Objects 2
Internet of Things vii, 1, 2, 53, 161
IoMT 20, 21, 24, 28, 29, 31–33, 39

K

Kaa (KaaIoT Technologies) 54
Kafka x, 154–159, 161

L

Legislation 21, 28, 29, 31–33
LoRaWAN – LoRa 8, 14

M

Magnetic Resonance Images (MRI) 26
MapReduce 140, 141, 143, 145–154, 159
Medical applications viii, 37, 38, 40–42, 45, 46, 114, 129
Medical imaging 20, 25, 28, 32
Medical video surveillance 27
Mindsphere (Siemens) 54

N

NFC: Near Field Communication 42, 45
NoSql 140–142

O

OFDM: Orthogonal Frequency Division Multiplexing 42

P

Pacemakers 64
Personalized medicine viii, 52
Pharmaceuticals viii, 51, 53, 59
Physical exercise 84–86, 88, 89, 102
Physical rehabilitation 88, 91, 123, 124
Positron Emission Tomography (PET) 26
Prediction 23, 25, 142
Prevention 23, 28, 39, 64, 121, 123, 127
Process management 2

R

Radio Frequency Identification 4
Rehabilitation ix, xi, 13, 14, 21, 39, 44, 83–88, 90–93, 98, 102, 103, 111, 114, 117, 118, 123–125
Remote medical assistance 9
Robotics xi, 20–23, 32

S

Security vii, xi, xii, 2, 3, 6, 14, 21, 28–30, 32, 33, 39, 42, 43, 46, 52, 55, 56, 58, 129, 142, 145
Segmentation 27
Sensors vii, ix, x, 1–4, 7, 10, 12, 14, 20, 28, 38–42, 44, 45, 51, 55, 65, 83–85, 89, 93, 94, 96, 98, 102, 112, 113, 130, 142, 161
Sonography 25
Spark x, 137, 140, 145–148, 154, 161
Stroke restoration 44
Swallowable pills 64

U

UWB: Ultra Wideband 42

W

Wearable antenna 38, 75–78
Wearable device viii, ix, 12, 24, 37–42, 45, 112, 114, 116, 118, 120, 129–131
Wearable health devices 38, 41, 43–46
Wearable sensors ix, 40, 41, 51, 83–85, 94, 112, 113
Wearable technology 40
Wireless Sensor Networks 2, 4, 28

Z

ZigBee 4, 14, 28, 42